Books should be returned on or before the
last date stamped below

12 NOV 05

- 7 SEP 2010

2 4 OCT 2012

- 1 MAR 2014

- 5 JUL 2019

1 9 JUL 2019

2 2 AUG 2019

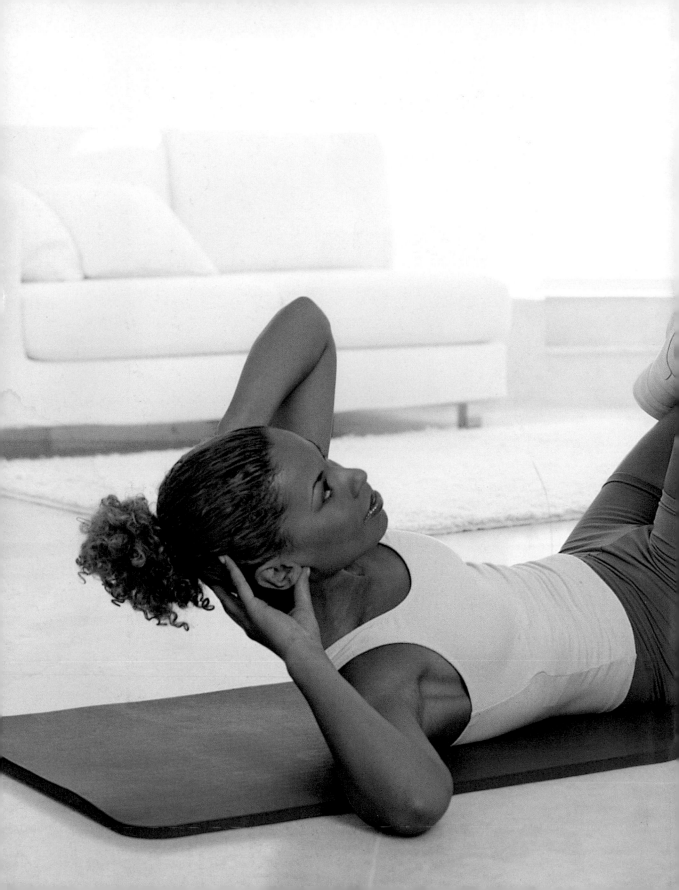

JOAN PAGANO
strength
training
for women

Tone up, burn calories, stay strong

LONDON, NEW YORK, MELBOURNE, MUNICH, and DELHI

For my mother, who has always been my inspiration

Senior Editor **Jennifer Jones**
Project Art Editor **Sara Robin**
Publishing Manager **Gillian Roberts**
Managing Art Editor **Marianne Markham**
Art Director **Carole Ash**
Publishing Director **Mary-Clare Jerram**
DTP Designer **Sonia Charbonnier**
Production Controller **Joanna Bull**

First published in Great Britain in 2005
by Dorling Kindersley Limited
80 Strand, London WC2R 0RL
Penguin Group (UK)

Always consult your doctor before starting a fitness
programme if you have any health concerns.

ISBN 1 4053 0643 2

Printed and bound by Tien Wah Press, Singapore
Colour reproduction by GRB, Italy

Discover more at
www.dk.com

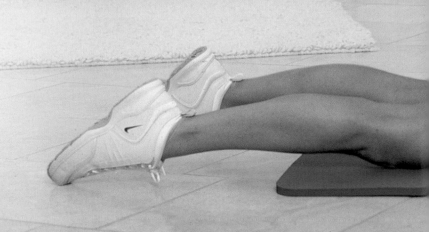

CONTENTS

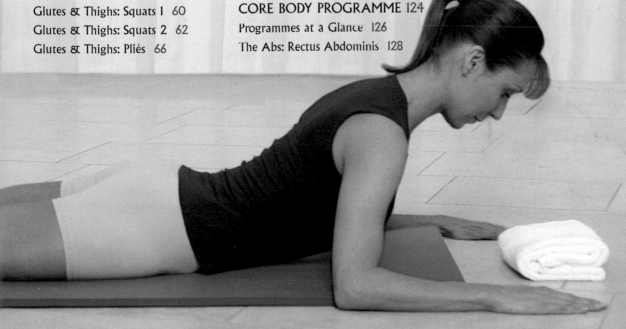

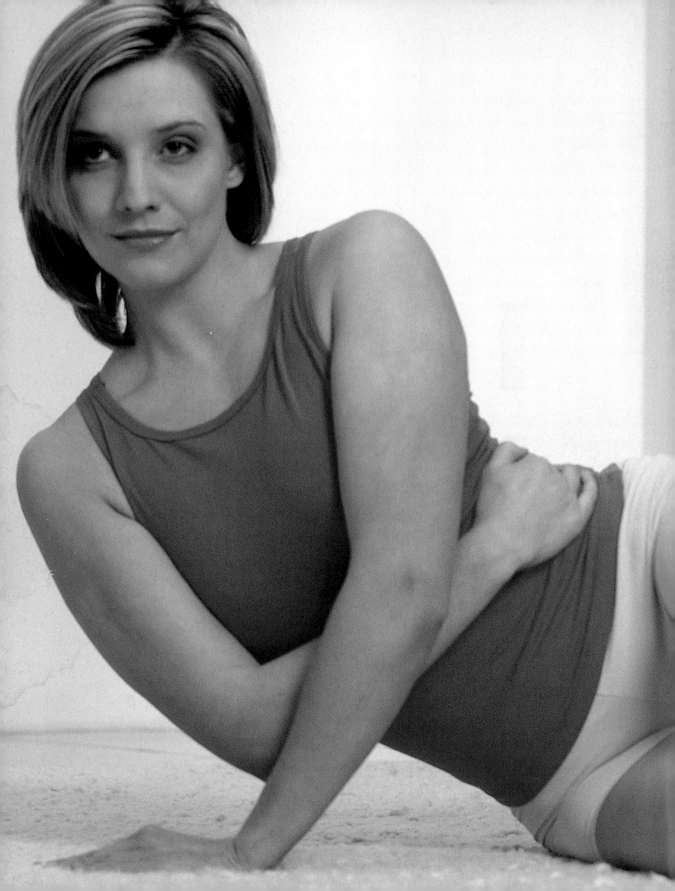

FIRST MOVES

Before you begin to exercise, you need to get your mind set

and your body ready. A little mental and physical preparation

work goes a long way to ensuring the success of your exercise

programme. Spend some time reviewing the contents of this

chapter, and enjoy the contemplation stage of making

positive change in your life. You have many exercise options

to choose from, and it is my intention to guide you through

the selection process to find the right options for you.

"Joan has trained me through my 30s, 40s, and now into my 50s; she has
worked occasionally with both of my children, as well as my parents, when
they were recovering from sports-related injuries. Sessions with Joan are one
of the highlights of my week (hard work but always enjoyable) and I credit
her with keeping me in good shape over the last 16 years." *Karen H.*

WHY LIFT WEIGHTS?

I was born with athletic abilities and you could say that fitness is in my bones. Nonetheless, there was a period of time in my life, roughly from ages 22 to 38, when I was sedentary until a friend shamed me into taking up yoga. This toned my musculature, but being tall, thin, and basically straight up and down, I wanted to take the next step and really sculpt some contours into my torso, arms, and legs. It was the beginning of a path that quickly led to a career in personal fitness training.

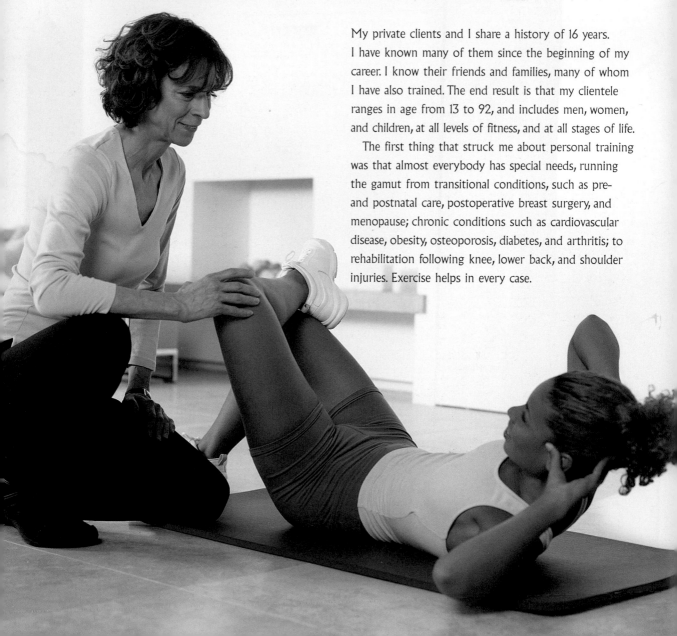

My private clients and I share a history of 16 years. I have known many of them since the beginning of my career. I know their friends and families, many of whom I have also trained. The end result is that my clientele ranges in age from 13 to 92, and includes men, women, and children, at all levels of fitness, and at all stages of life.

The first thing that struck me about personal training was that almost everybody has special needs, running the gamut from transitional conditions, such as pre- and postnatal care, postoperative breast surgery, and menopause; chronic conditions such as cardiovascular disease, obesity, osteoporosis, diabetes, and arthritis; to rehabilitation following knee, lower back, and shoulder injuries. Exercise helps in every case.

Women's health I did not pick my areas of special interest in women's health issues as much as they picked me. One client who had had breast surgery made such dramatic progress in her fitness programme that she felt there must be other women who would benefit too. With her encouragement and with the supervision of Dr. David Hidalgo, then Chief of Plastic and Reconstructive Surgery at Memorial Sloan–Kettering Cancer Center in New York City, I pioneered exercise guidelines for postoperative breast surgery.

My work with cancer survivors continued at SHARE, a self-help group for women with breast and/or ovarian cancer. Their concerns about menopause – both because they are of menopausal age and also because their treatments may induce an early and abrupt menopause – prompted me to study how exercise can help manage the side effects of this transition and, in particular, how exercise can help fight osteoporosis.

RESISTANCE TRAINING FOR LIFE

Most people are familiar with the term strength training, but they may not be aware that it is a method of resistance training, a broader category that also includes endurance training. Resistance training (also referred to as weight training or weight lifting) is the technique of applying resistance to the muscles to stimulate growth (hypertrophy) of the muscle fibres and increase circulation to them. Skeletal muscle is composed of two different kinds of fibres: slow twitch and fast twitch. The body uses slow-twitch fibres for prolonged endurance work, while fast-twitch fibres provide strength and power for higher-intensity demands.

Depending on the training method you use, you can develop both strength and endurance in the muscles. Strength is measured by the amount of force you can produce with one all-out effort; endurance by the number of times you can sustain a muscular contraction before you fatigue. Strength allows you to lift a case of baby formula into the boot of a car, while endurance allows you to carry heavy shopping home.

Young adulthood As early as age 25, you may begin to lose muscle mass and strength without being aware of it. Subtle changes begin to occur in your body composition that are not reflected on the bathroom scales. Even if you maintain your weight perfectly over time, if you do not lift weights your lean body mass begins to decline and your body fat increases.

Body composition is the "quality" of your weight as opposed to the "quantity" of your weight measured by the scale. You can gauge your body-fat status roughly by the fit of a favourite pair of jeans. Half a kilogram (1lb) of fat takes up more space than 0.5kg (1lb) of muscle, so as you lose fat you literally shrink. (Think of the meat on display at a butcher's: a 1.5-kg/3-lb beef roast is small compared to 1.5kg/3lb of fat.)

Lifting weights will sculpt the contours of your body. You will have a flatter tummy, shapelier arms, firmer legs, and you will look great in a little black dress. But the benefits don't stop there. Being strong gives you a sense of empowerment. It means that you can be more independent and self-reliant. One of the reasons I started weight training was that after my divorce I couldn't count on anyone else to help me move furniture around my flat, or to carry my suitcase when I went on holiday.

When it comes to being physically active, weight training strengthens the muscles and joints so that you can increase the intensity and duration of cardiovascular work, enhancing your aerobic workouts and sports activities. It will make you more resilient to injury, and less likely to suffer poor posture and back pain. It can help prepare you for childbirth and also help you recover your prepregnancy weight, strength, and flexibility levels.

The middle years As you approach middle age (35–50), strength training keeps you lean by building muscle. Lean body mass has a higher resting metabolic rate than fat, burning more calories as you breathe, digest food, even as you sleep. I consider the middle years to

OSTEOPOROSIS AND FRACTURES: THE RISKS

Osteoporosis is a preventable and treatable condition, but because it is a silent disease with no apparent symptoms until a fracture occurs, many women are not being diagnosed in the early stages of the disease when therapy can be effective. Osteoporosis does not just affect older women. Younger woman can also suffer from osteoporosis, and in my opinion should seek professional advice based on the number of risk factors they have (see below). The seeds of this disease are planted in childhood and adolescence, although it may not manifest until decades later. The more risk factors, the greater the risk for fracture.

Risk factors based on personal history
- Female
- Small, thin frame
- Incidence of low-impact fracture
- Family history of fracture in parent or sibling, and/or history of osteoporosis
- Caucasian race
- Early menopause (before age 45)
- Advanced age
- Poor health/frailty/dementia

Risk factors based on lifestyle considerations
- Current low bone-mineral density (BMD)
- Low body weight i.e. less than 57.5kg (127lb)
- Low oestrogen levels
- Amenorrhoea (loss of normal menstrual period, when not pregnant)
- Low lifetime calcium intake
- Low lifetime physical activity
- Current smoker
- Excessive use of alcohol (more than 2 drinks per day)

Risk factors due to medical conditions and medications
- Eating disorders (e.g. anorexia nervosa), past or present
- Long-term use of steroids and other drugs used to treat asthma, lupus, rheumatoid arthritis, epilepsy, bipolar disorder, and breast cancer
- Thyroid and pituitary disorders
- Diseases that interfere with the absorption of calcium e.g. coeliac disease and liver disease

be a maintenance phase. Research shows that much of what we consider the ageing process – the loss of strength, stamina, bone density, balance, and flexibility – is actually due to inactivity. A well-designed exercise programme that includes weight training will impact your weight, health, fitness, and well-being for decades to come. Weight training helps reduce your risk for cardiovascular disease, diabetes, and osteoporosis in later life (and helps manage these diseases if they develop).

The menopausal years In the menopausal years (about 50-plus), hormonal changes cause some loss of muscle with accompanying weight gain, but again, you can keep this to a minimum with weight training.

As we age, we start to slow down and need help lifting things. The fast-twitch muscle fibres shrink in size, causing not only a loss of muscle mass, but also a loss of power. Restoring muscle restores your strength and energy levels.

Strengthening the muscles benefits the bones as well. As you work with weights, you overload the muscles, which respond by getting stronger. The pull of the muscle on the bone has a similar effect in strengthening the bones, offsetting age-related bone loss and even regaining some lost bone.

The later years With advancing age (70-plus), weight training creates stability, especially in the large muscles of the legs, which can help your balance and walking ability. Studies show that you are never too old to begin a weight-training programme and that lifting weights can improve your quality of life even into your 80s and 90s. The improvement in strength, balance, and bone density reduces your risk of falling and fracturing a bone. Strong people are more active and self-sufficient. Your "functional independence" is measured by your ability to perform all of your day-to-day activities, which together comprise a lifestyle. As long as you maintain a young functional age, then your chronological age is truly just a number.

OSTEOPOROSIS

Current research on osteoporosis is focused on how strength training can prevent and treat this condition. Osteoporosis – which means literally "porous bones" – is a bone-thinning disease caused by a loss of mineral (primarily calcium) that weakens the bone structure. The bone becomes vulnerable to fracture.

About 40 per cent of all fractures occur in the spine, resulting in a loss of height and a stooped posture. About 25 per cent of fractures occur in the hip, most often in the upper part of the thighbone (the femur). The effect of a hip fracture is particularly debilitating and life-altering. About half of the people affected are not able to walk unassisted again. Fifteen per cent of fractures occur at the wrist, often the result of an outstretched hand to break a fall.

The ultimate goal of exercise for osteoporosis is to reduce the risk of falls and hip fractures. It is clear that strength not only helps conserve bone mass, but also maintains muscle mass and improves balance, both of which help prevent falls. Exercise has a dramatic effect on the growing skeleton, which is why it is essential for children to be physically active. Once the skeleton stops growing, the effect of exercise on the bone is more modest. If you do not develop adequate bone-mineral density at an early age, your risk of osteoporosis increases in the postmenopausal years. However, some bone lost through inactivity may be restored and major bone losses can be prevented before ages 30 to 35.

After menopause, research suggests that exercise alone cannot prevent bone loss, but it can help preserve bone. If you are 50-plus, and postmenopausal, you should ask your physician about having a bone density test as a baseline. In the first three to seven years after menopause, you may lose bone at an accelerated rate before it levels off to a more modest decline. Your doctor may recommend drug therapy during this time, in addition to adequate calcium intake and appropriate exercise. It is vital to continue with resistance training as well as balance and stretching exercises.

EXERCISE GUIDELINES AND RESTRICTIONS

From 18–35:
The goal is to achieve the highest peak bone mass. Exercise should maximize the load to the bones with a progressive programme of:
- High-impact exercise, defined as activities in which both feet are off the ground at the same time, as in running, skipping, and high-impact aerobic dance; also sports like basketball, volleyball, and gymnastics.
- High-intensity weight lifting, as in the Bone-Building Programme in this book (see p19), using free weights ranging from 2–7kg (5–15lb).

From 35–50:
The goal is to maintain bone mass, offset or reduce bone loss, and improve your coordination and balance:
- Follow the guidelines above, and focus on strengthening the bony sites most vulnerable to fracture: the thighbone, the spine, and the wrist.
- Add balance training, e.g. standing on one leg (see p26); stability-ball exercises (see p27).

From 50-plus and post-menopausal:
Follow the guidelines for ages 35–50. Focus on strengthening the muscles of the leg for stability. If you have osteoporosis, follow the guidelines below.

Exercise restrictions for osteoporosis:
The goal is to protect the spine and avoid falls:
- Do not jar the spine (avoid impact exercise).
- Avoid spinal flexion (forward bending) in all positions, e.g. crunches (see pp128–129).
- Do not perform spinal rotations (twisting the torso), e.g. Side Twist with Ball (p131).
- Avoid flexion with rotation, e.g. Side Crunch (p130).
- Do not perform jarring movements with rotation, e.g. tennis, golf, bowling. (Note: if you want to continue with your sport, consult with a physical therapist for advice on biomechanics to protect the spine.)
- In weight lifting, start with lighter weights, i.e. the Shaping and Toning Programme (see p17), and work up to more challenging resistance and fewer repetitions (see Bone-Building Programme, p19).
- Check with your doctor for approval of your exercise choices and weight limitations.

TEST YOUR FITNESS

Before you start your weight-training programme (or any exercise programme), you must check that it is safe for you to begin. Take the Par-Q questionnaire on the opposite page, and if you are in any doubt about the state of your health, please see your doctor before becoming more physically active. The three fitness tests below will help you to establish your current level of fitness and provide you with a way of measuring your progress over the next weeks and months.

MUSCULAR FITNESS

One way to measure muscular fitness is to count how many repetitions you can perform, or how many seconds you can hold a contraction. To see how you measure up, do the three exercises below, which will assess your muscular endurance in the lower, middle, and upper body. Write down your results, make a note of the date, and after three months of training, repeat the assessment.

When you reassess yourself, perform the same version of the exercise.

If you are just beginning to exercise, or coming back to it after a long absence, you may prefer to perform your first assessment after two or three months of exercising on a regular basis. Before attempting the exercises below, warm up first by walking around or moving your arms and legs briskly for 5 minutes.

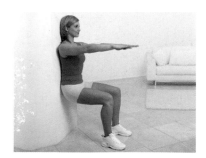

Lower Body
Wall Squat (pp38–39)
Slide down until your thighs are parallel to the floor and hold the position for as long as you can. (If you cannot slide all the way down, go as far as you can.)

Your score

Excellent	90 seconds or more
Good	60 seconds
Fair	30 seconds
Poor	less than 30 seconds

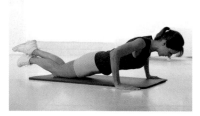

Upper Body
Half Press-Up (p44)
Count how many Half Press-Ups you can do consecutively without a rest. If you cannot perform the Half Press-Up, do the Wall Press-Up (p42) or the Diagonal Press-Up (p43).

Your score

Excellent	20 reps or more
Good	15–19 reps
Fair	10–14 reps
Poor	10 reps or less

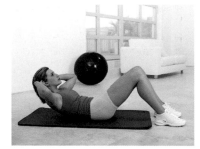

Middle Body
Crunch with Scoop (p129)
Count how many crunches you can do consecutively without resting. This is not a full sit-up. Lift your head and shoulders no higher than 30 degrees off the mat.

Your score

Excellent	50 reps or more
Good	35–49 reps
Fair	20–34 reps
Poor	20 reps or less

PAR-Q AND YOU   A questionnaire for people aged 15 to 69

Physical Activity Readiness Questionnaire – Par-Q (revised 2002)

Regular physical activity is fun and healthy, and increasingly more people are starting to become more active every day. Being more active is very safe for most people. However, some people should check with their doctor before they start becoming much more physically active.

If you are planning to become much more physically active than you are now, start by answering the seven questions in the box below. If you are between the ages of 15 and 69, the PAR-Q will tell you if you should check with your doctor before you start. If you are over 69 years of age, and you are not used to being very active, check with your doctor.

Common sense is your best guide when you answer these questions. Please read the questions carefully and answer each one honestly: check YES or NO.

YES   NO

☐ ☐ **1** Has your doctor ever said that you have a heart condition <u>and</u> that you should only do physical activity recommended by a doctor?

☐ ☐ **2** Do you feel pain in your chest when you do physical activity?

☐ ☐ **3** In the past month, have you had chest pain when you were not doing physical activity?

☐ ☐ **4** Do you lose your balance because of dizziness or do you ever lose consciousness?

YES   NO

☐ ☐ **5** Do you have a bone or joint problem (for example, back, knee or hip) that could be made worse by a change in your physical activity?

☐ ☐ **6** Is your doctor currently prescribing drugs (for example, water pills) for your blood pressure or heart condition?

☐ ☐ **7** Do you know of <u>any other reason</u> why you should not do physical activity?

If you answered YES to one or more questions

Talk with your doctor by phone or in person BEFORE you start becoming much more physically active or BEFORE you have a fitness appraisal.
Tell your doctor about the PAR-Q and which questions you answered YES.
• You may be able to do any activity you want – as long as you start slowly and build up gradually. Or, you may need to restrict your activities to those which are safe for you. Talk with your doctor about the kinds of activities you wish to participate in and follow his/her advice.
• Find out which community programmes are safe and helpful for you.

If you answered NO to all questions

If you answered NO honestly to <u>all</u> PAR-Q questions, you can be reasonably sure that you can:
• start becoming much more physically active – begin slowly and build up gradually. This is the safest and easiest way to go.
• take part in a fitness appraisal – this is an excellent way to determine your basic fitness so that you can plan the best way for you to live actively. It is also highly recommended that you have your blood pressure evaluated. If your reading is over 144/94, talk with your doctor before you start becoming much more physically active.

DELAY BECOMING MUCH MORE ACTIVE:
• if you are not feeling well because of a temporary illness such as a cold or a fever – wait until you feel better; or
• if you are or may be pregnant – talk to your doctor before you start becoming more active.

PLEASE NOTE:
If your health changes so that you then answer YES to any of the above questions, tell your fitness or health professional. Ask whether you should change your physical activity plan.

YOUR TRAINING PROGRAMME

The principles of training will guide you in the development of your exercise programme and help you to determine which methods will deliver the results you want. Keep this in mind as you look at the different factors of the training session (*pp16–18*). To achieve your fitness goals, you need to make the right choices about exercise on a daily basis and assess your progress regularly. The SMART system of goal-setting (*pp18–19*) will help you to stay on course.

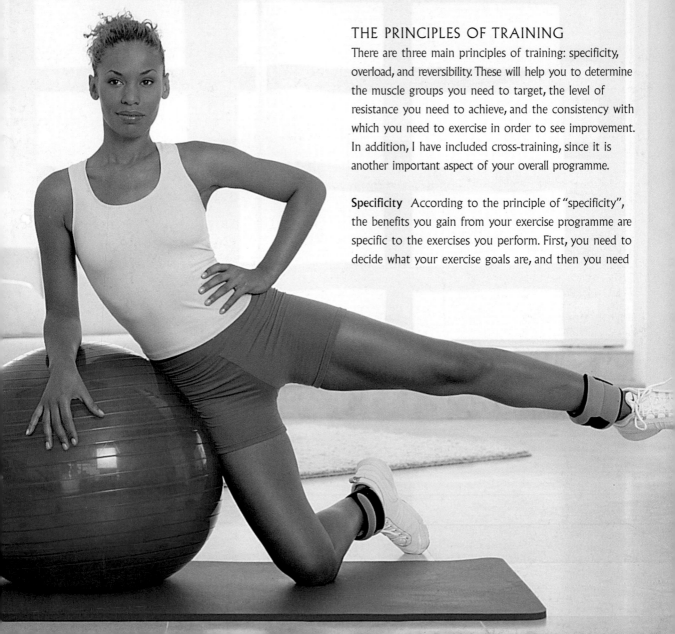

THE PRINCIPLES OF TRAINING

There are three main principles of training: specificity, overload, and reversibility. These will help you to determine the muscle groups you need to target, the level of resistance you need to achieve, and the consistency with which you need to exercise in order to see improvement. In addition, I have included cross-training, since it is another important aspect of your overall programme.

Specificity According to the principle of "specificity", the benefits you gain from your exercise programme are specific to the exercises you perform. First, you need to decide what your exercise goals are, and then you need to establish which methods of training will support them. For example, if you want to maintain bone density, you will need to do strength-training exercises that are site-specific because bone deposition occurs only at the site of stress, where the muscle pulls on the bone. So you need to be careful to include all the major areas of the skeleton in your workout, and target the specific sites that commonly fracture with weak bones: the hip (upper thighbone), the spine, and the wrist.

Overload The principle of "overload" dictates that for any physiological system (i.e. the muscles, the skeleton, the heart, and the lungs) to improve its function, it must be exposed to a load larger than normal. For strong bones, it means that the skeleton must encounter forces greater than those it sustains on a day-to-day basis. Obviously this is very individual. If you have been bedridden or are a "professional sitter", then simply doing the "4 for Life" exercises (see pp38–51) constitutes overload. If you are already an active person, then you need to look at exercises that offer more stimulus to the bones, such as the Shaping and Toning Programme (see p17) or the Bone-Building Programme (see p19).

Reversibility The principle of "reversibility" states that the benefits of exercise are transient and that they are lost with disuse. The effects of disuse on the bone are dramatic, as shown in studies on space flight (in the absence of gravity), bed rest, and paralysis. Unless the bone is continually subjected to stress, the breakdown process outruns the building process and the bones become porous and weak.

Cross-training This has important implications for bone health. Because bone loading is site-specific, you need to do a range of exercises to stimulate the bones with diverse patterns of stress. For instance, if you are already doing a weight-bearing aerobic activity such as walking, which will impact the hip, you should add resistance exercises for the upper body. It is important to vary

MYTHS OF STRENGTH TRAINING

Myth 1: Lifting weights will make you bulk up.
Truth: Only if you have high levels of testosterone and use very heavy weights. Most women lack the necessary hormones and strength to build muscle mass. Female body builders are genetically predisposed to build big muscles; they also follow rigorous exercise and diet regimes to maximize their muscle size. The average woman who lifts weights actually shrinks in body size by losing fat and shaping the muscles.

Myth 2: You shouldn't lift weights if you are an older adult, overweight, or out of shape.
Truth: Not so! Weight training can help you rejuvenate, lose weight, and shape up. Begin with 4–6 simple exercises that are manageable (see 4 for Life, pp38-51) and gradually progress by increasing the level of difficulty and adding exercises.

Myth 3: A thin person does not need to build lean body mass by lifting weights.
Truth: Appearances are deceiving when it comes to body composition, and being thin is no guarantee that you are lean (see p9). Without weight training, you steadily lose muscle and gain fat as you age.

Myth 4: Certain weight-training exercises can help you spot reduce.
Truth: You can spot *strengthen* and shape a body area, but fat belongs to the whole body and needs to be reduced all over, through expending more calories (aerobic exercise and weight training) than you consume. If you want to balance out your proportions, for example if you have broad hips, use the Shaping and Toning Programme (see p17) for your lower body and the Bone-Building Programme (see p19) for the upper body. High-repetition training will keep the hips trim; while using heavier weights to strengthen the upper body can make your hips look more in balance.

Myth 5: Aerobic activities, not weight training, are the most efficient type of exercise to lose weight.
Truth: Losing weight requires a balanced exercise programme of aerobic exercise to burn calories and weight training to speed up the metabolism.

A walking programme is weight-bearing on the hips and legs, but can leave the rest of your body undeveloped. Be sure to add exercises with weights for the upper body.

OTHER TRAINING FACTORS

One of the most important training factors is that because we are all different, everyone's training needs will vary. Your exercise programme must take into account who you are, what your goals are, what you like, what works for you, and how you respond.

If you are just beginning, it is best to start with a simple exercise plan on which you can build, and which will provide the baseline plan to which you can always return. Choose between eight and ten exercises and do them consistently for two to three weeks to make sure that you don't experience discomfort anywhere. Squats and lunges, for instance, are both great exercises, but they can cause problems if you have weak knees.

It is important to start gently and progress gradually. It takes time to learn to coordinate the movements gracefully and to develop body awareness of the proper form of the exercises. Your muscles need to adjust gradually to the new demands and starting gradually helps to minimize any muscle soreness. In addition, the tissue that connects muscles and bones (tendons and ligaments) needs time to adapt. Gradual conditioning of the connective tissue strengthens the joints and prevents injuries such as torn ligaments and tendonitis. Even if you are naturally strong and capable of lifting heavy weights, if you haven't previously trained with weights, you need to protect your joints by building up slowly. The older you are, the more careful you need to be to allow for these adjustments when you begin to lift weights. Patience pays off in the long run.

your walking route to include hills and steps, adding intervals of increased speed or jogging, if appropriate. Upper-body exercises should include strengthening exercises with resistance, as well as "straightening" exercises, such as back extensions (*see pp46–49*), to improve posture. If you enjoy swimming and biking, which are weight-supported activities, make sure you add some weight-bearing exercises for the hips and legs, such as squats (*pp38–41, 60–64*) and lunges (*pp68–70*), to create a well-rounded exercise programme.

Exercise selection and order Your entire programme should include a minimum of eight to ten separate exercises that work the major muscle groups (*see pp20–21*).

You should work in the order of large to small muscle groups so as not to fatigue the smaller muscles first. The smaller muscles help stabilize the larger ones, but if you exhaust them first they cannot support the larger muscles in their work, making it more difficult to complete the exercises.

Mode of resistance Calisthenics are exercises that use body weight alone (a shift in body weight can increase or decrease the level of resistance). External forms of resistance include free weights, machines, weighted bars and balls, stretch bands, and resistance tubes.

Machines support your body in the correct position and, generally, allow you to lift more weight than if you were using free weights. I have included several machine exercises to complement the at-home programme. Unfortunately, the machines do not provide a good fit for every body and, if the settings are not compatible with your height and limb length, they can cause joint injuries. Also, they do not always offer a light enough weight that you can work if you are just beginning to train.

Free weights, on the other hand, highlight imbalances (asymmetries) in the body, since you use them with individual limbs; they can be an effective tool for correcting these imbalances and for bringing the body into alignment. They make weight lifting more like a sport by challenging your balance, coordination, and full-body stabilization. The optimal formula is a combination of calisthenics, free weights, and machines.

Frequency and duration You need to do a minimum of two weight-training sessions per week to achieve the desired training effects, and no muscle should be worked more than three times in one week. Allow one day of rest in between working each muscle group, since the repair and recovery of the muscle fibres is as important as the stress to the development of the muscle. If you want to weight train every day, you can do a "split-body" routine: upper body one day, lower body the next. If you want to work the upper body every day, you can alternate pushing exercises with pulling exercises: e.g. chest, shoulders, and triceps on day one; back and biceps on day two.

The length of your session will vary according to how many exercises and sets you choose. Sessions with my clients are about 45 minutes long. Programmes of more than an hour tend to have high dropout rates.

SHAPING AND TONING PROGRAMME

If you are just beginning to exercise, or are starting again after a long absence, it is best to start with exercises that use your own body weight as resistance. The 4 for Life chapter (pp28–55) gives you four classics: the squat, the press-up, the back extension, and the pelvic tilt. When you are ready, move on to the exercises in the rest of the book and follow the shaping and toning guidelines in the weights and repetitions boxes for the exercises. This gives you an endurance-training programme using lighter weights and higher repetitions (12–15 reps).

Choosing weights

If you are an older adult or very out of shape, start with even lighter weights than those recommended in the shaping and toning guidelines. You can use something from your kitchen cabinet like a pair of 0.5kg (1lb) soup cans. If you are healthy and without joint pain, start with a pair of 1–2kg (3–5lb) free weights. Concentrate on using proper form, maintaining your posture, and coordinating the movement with your breathing. Inhale first, then exhale slowly as you lift the weight, controlling the pace with your breath. When you can complete 1 set of 10 reps, rest and repeat.

When you can do 2 sets of 10 reps without stress, move into the full Shaping and Toning Programme. This trains the muscle to contract repeatedly before fatiguing, as when you carry a tired toddler home from playing in the park. Use weights that you can lift 12–15 times in good form, but the last few should be somewhat hard. This is generally a safe protocol that will train and shape the muscles without injuring the joints.

Maintenance programme

To maintain your improvement in endurance without increasing the resistance, you can add more sets, which will continue your endurance training without developing additional strength. Periodically, you should change the exercises and the order that you do them so that you keep your muscles "alert". To progress to strength training, see the Bone-Building Programme on p19. However, the strength-training programme may not be suitable for everyone (see Cautions on p19).

Repetitions and sets Repetitions (reps) are the number of times you repeat one particular exercise, lifting and lowering the weight. In some exercises you have a choice to lift the weights simultaneously, both arms together, or to alternate sides, lifting one arm or leg and then the other. If the exercise calls for 12 reps, then you need to do 12 reps with each side. Doing all reps on one side first provides more of an overload to the muscles involved; alternating sides provides a minirest to one side between reps. You should always begin work with your weaker side in order to give it priority and not to overstrengthen the dominant side, only to find you cannot finish the same number of reps on the weaker side.

Speed of repetitions You should lift a weight (or weights) on a count of 2, and lower on a count of 4. Muscles build by a cycle of microdamage (lifting weights) and repair of the muscle fibres (your rest days). As the muscle repairs, it gets stronger. The lowering phase of muscular contraction, when you resist the pull of gravity, appears to be more critical than the lifting phase in the building cycle, which is another reason to emphasize it by slowing that phase of the repetition.

Range of motion For optimal development, you should work each muscle through its full range of motion. It is important to keep tension in the muscle throughout the entire movement, and not to relax the part of the body being worked after the lowering phase. Also, use caution not to "crank the joints" by hyperextending them at the end range of motion, since this causes unnecessary wear and tear.

Intensity You should work to the point of volitional fatigue ("I can't do any more"). There are different methods to achieve muscular failure. You can overload the muscle with the amount of weight that you use, with the number of reps, or with a combination of both. I sometimes like to end a weight-training set by using light weights or calisthenics (using body weight), such as a press-up (*pp42–45*) or the Wall Squat (*pp38–39*), to bring a muscle to fatigue.

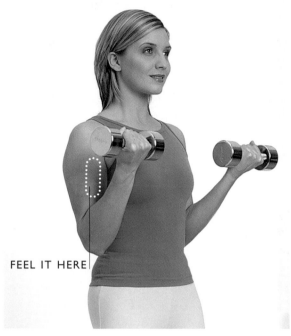

FEEL IT HERE

Work muscles in full range of motion. When you do a biceps curl, for example, extend the elbow fully as you lower the weight and flex the elbow fully as you lift it. The Feel It Here symbol helps you to focus on working the proper muscle. Put your mind on it and give an additional squeeze as you feel the muscle contract with the movement.

SET YOURSELF UP FOR SUCCESS

A little advance planning in terms of your exercise goals and expectations can go a long way to keeping you on track. Goal-setting is one of the best ways to stay motivated to exercise. If you have a clear purpose, you are more likely to persevere. Experts in the field of self-improvement often recommend the SMART system of goal-setting, which states that goals must be Specific, Measurable, Action-oriented, Realistic, and Timed.

Specific "Wanting to get in shape" is not specific enough. What exactly do you want to accomplish? Reduce fat, improve muscle tone, increase bone density? Once you are clear about what your goals are, you can choose exercises that will support them.

Measurable Unless your goal is measurable, you have no way of knowing if you accomplished it. Specific goals are measurable. Reducing fat can be measured by fitting into your favourite jeans. Muscle tone can be measured by endurance exercises, such as a squat, a press-up, and a crunch (*see Test Your Fitness, pp12–13*). Bone density is measured by a bone density test.

Action-oriented Have a written action plan that breaks your long-term goal into weekly targets. This gives you both the satisfaction of meeting short-term goals and a regular opportunity to assess whether your goals are reasonable. For example, do your goals fit your lifestyle? Your schedule? Your work and family obligations? If your action plan appears to be unrealistic, you need to adjust it. Remember, it usually takes four to six weeks to change old habits.

Realistic Don't be a casualty of unrealistic goals. People often become disillusioned and stop exercising when they don't get their imagined results, such as in spot reducing. Give your goals the reality test. For example, are they in sync with your body type? If you are a muscular woman with large bones, you will never be rail thin. Do they match your personal preferences? If you hate a particular exercise, you won't do it, so find one you do like. Focus on what you enjoy.

Timed Setting a target date gives you the motivation to stick with an exercise programme for the long term. Without a target date, you have not fully committed to your programme. You must allow enough time to achieve your goal. It is not realistic to expect to lose 9kg (20lb) in one month; a more realistic goal is four to five months.

BONE-BUILDING PROGRAMME

Once you are doing the Shaping and Toning programme (see p17) on a regular basis (two to three times per week for four to eight weeks), you are ready to follow the bone-building guidelines in the weights and repetitions boxes for the exercises. This gives you a strength-training programme using heavier weights and fewer repetitions (8–12 reps). This trains the muscle to produce more force, making it easier to lift something heavy without straining or to power up a steep incline. The Bone-Building Programme will help to build bone in young skeletons and conserve bone and muscle mass in mature skeletons.

Improvement phase

To maintain your new level of strength, add more sets (up to 3). When this programme becomes easy for you, initiate a new cycle of improvement by increasing the number of repetitions to an endurance level (12–15 reps). Periodically change the exercises and the order in which you do them to stimulate the muscles.

After a lay off, start with 50–75 per cent less resistance than your previous level, and build up gradually.

Cautions

You should not exercise with heavy weights if you have hypertension; a history of neck, shoulder, elbow, hip, or knee injury; or carpel tunnel syndrome or any other wrist problems. Consult your physician and/or physical therapist if you have a history of back problems.

It is also imperative that you address the whole body. If you have a weak lower back or a tricky knee, don't ignore it while you work on strengthening other muscles. Get a professional diagnosis and ask for guidance in what exercises are appropriate for strengthening weak areas.

Choosing weights: exercise caution

Some experts recommend lifting very heavy weights for a bone-building programme. What I have learned from my clients is that there is no one workout appropriate for everybody, and that the upper limits vary not only from person to person, but also throughout the body. Increasing the weights may trigger problems in the neck, shoulder, elbow, lower back, or knees. You may be able to handle heavier weights in some muscle groups, but not in others. Finding the right weights is a process of careful discovery.

ANATOMY OF AN EXERCISE

A whole-body training programme should include a minimum of 8–10 separate exercises that work the major muscle groups. Use this index to guide you in picking exercises from each group. Ideally, start with the largest muscles and work down to the smallest (*see box opposite*).

CHEST
Pectorals
Press-ups series, pp42–45
Modified pull-over, p103
Chest flye, p104
Chest press, p105
Chest press on chest-press machine, p107
Chest flye on pec-dec machine, p108

ARMS
Biceps
Alternating biceps curl, p116
Biceps "21s", p117

ABDOMEN
Pelvic-tilt series, pp50–51
Plank series, pp138–141
Obliques
Side crunch, p130
Side twist with ball, p131
Rectus abdominis
Reverse crunch, p128
Crunch with scoop, p129
Crunch on ball, p129
Transversus abdominis
Dead-bug series, pp132–135

FOREARM, WRISTS
Strengthening the wrists, pp142–143

OUTER THIGH
Hip abductor
Outer-thigh lift, p80
Outer-thigh lift on ball, p81
Seated hip abduction on hip-abductor machine, p83
Side-stepping with tube, p84

FRONT OF THIGH
Quadriceps
Pliés, pp34, 66–67
Squats series, pp38–41, 60–62
Leg-press machine series, pp63–64
Lunges series, pp68–70
Knee extensions, pp72–73

LOWER LEG, SHIN AND ANKLES
Calf raise on leg-press machine, p65
Strengthening the ankles, pp144–145

SHOULDER
Deltoid
Diagonal press-up, p43
Horizontal abduction, p52
Standing front raise, p110
Side-lying lateral raise, p111
Side-lying reverse flye, p112
"Ys" and "Ts" on ball, pp114–115

Rotator cuff
External rotation, p53
Side-lying external rotation, p113

ARMS
Triceps
Lying triceps extension, p105
Triceps-kickback series, p118–119
One-arm triceps push-down, p120
Side-lying triceps press-up, p121

BUTTOCKS
Gluteals/Glutes
Pliés, pp34, 66–67
Squats series, pp38–41, 60–62
Leg-press machine series, pp63–64
Lunges series, pp68–70
Bent-leg lift, p74
Raised glute squeeze, p76
Ball bridge, p77

BACK OF THIGH
Hamstrings
Straight-leg lift, p75
Ball bridge, p77
Leg curl on ball, p77
Hamstring curl on prone
leg-curl machine, p78

THE MAJOR MUSCLE GROUPS

Try to work in the order of large to small muscle groups, as follows: **Hips and thighs** (gluteals, quadriceps, hamstrings, and hip adductors and abductors); **Back** (latissimus dorsi, rhomboids, trapezius, and erector spinae); **Chest** (pectorals); **Shoulders** (deltoid); **Arms** (biceps and triceps); and **Abdomen** (rectus abdominis, transversus abdominis, and the obliques).

BACK
Serratus anterior
Scapular thrust, p102
Scapular thrust on chest press, p106

Rhomboids and Trapezius
Posture-plus series, pp52–53
Upper-back row, p95
Scapular retraction, p96
Upper-back row, p97
Reverse flye on pec-dec machine, p109

Latissimus dorsi
One-arm row, p94
Bent-over lat row, p95
Lat row, p96
Shoulder extension, p97
Lat pull-down series, pp98–101

Erector spinae
Back extensions series, pp46–49
Back extension on leg-curl machine, p79
Arm-and-leg-lift series, pp136–137

INNER THIGH
Hip adductor
Pliés, pp34, 66–67
Inner-thigh lift, p81
Scissors with tubes, p85
Seated hip adduction on
hip-adductor machine, p83

LOWER LEG, CALF
Calf raise on leg-press machine, p65
Calf raise, p71

EQUIPMENT

To begin training, I recommend two pairs of free weights (also called hand weights or dumbbells), either 1kg (3lb) and 2kg (5lb), or 2kg (5lb) and 4kg (8lb), depending on your starting level; one pair of 1kg (3lb) ankle weights; three 1.2m (4ft) long stretch bands of varying resistance, and an exercise mat. You can also be creative in borrowing household items such as soup cans for a very basic starting level of resistance (*see p17*); thick carpet can take the place of a mat for many of the exercises.

WHAT TO WEAR

Wear comfortable clothing that you can move in. Some of my clients prefer form-fitting clothing because it makes it easier to monitor body alignment doing the exercises. Others prefer loose-fitting clothing that is not so revealing. In any case, the fabric should "breathe" to assist the body's cooling system. You should have supportive shoes such as cross-trainers that allow for movement in a variety of directions. Running shoes are not advisable because they are designed primarily for moving only forwards and backwards.

SPECIFIC RECOMMENDATIONS

My preferences in equipment choices are based on quality, economy, and safety of use.

Free weights These are usually solid metal covered in grey enamel, chrome, vinyl, or neoprene (which contains latex). Enamel or chrome coating may chip and flake over time, presenting a risk in use. The vinyl and neoprene coatings eliminate this risk, come in bright colours, and are nicer to hold. I prefer neoprene-covered free weights because they do not become slippery with sweat. Free weights are most widely available in weight increments of .05-, 1-, 2-kg, 3-kg, and so on, or 1-, 2-, 3-lb, 4-lb, and so on. The conversions in this book, therefore, are only approximate.

Ankle or cuff weights They are either nonadjustable or adjustable. One kilogram (3lb) is generally a good all-purpose denomination, but the adjustable pairs (up

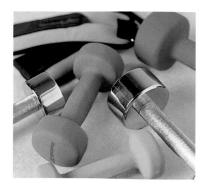

Free weights come in a variety of finishes. Your weights should be comfortable to hold and easy to use. Ankle weights should fasten with minimum fuss.

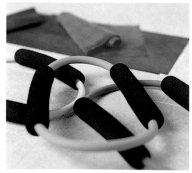

Different coloured bands and tubes indicate different levels of resistance. Foam handles make them easier to hold and offer cushioning if you use them against your legs.

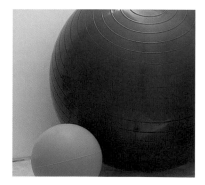

Balls come in a variety of sizes and weights. Large stability balls are great for balance training. Weighted balls in small and medium sizes offer another type of resistance.

to 2kg/5lb or 4.5kg/10lb per leg) offer more versatility. An additional feature to look for is the length of the tail or closure. I prefer a 1kg (3lb) nonadjustable cuff weight with a long touch-fastener tail because it fits above the knee as well as at the ankle or wrist. If you have any conditions in your hands, such as arthritis, that might prevent you from holding a free weight, all of these weights offer an alternative.

Mats Exercise mats are available in different densities of foam that either fold or roll up. Of the foldable exercise mats, I prefer the dense foam, which is stiff to touch but surprisingly resilient to use. Of the roll-up exercise mats, I prefer a soft durable foam mat (*see Resources, p159*) because it offers comfortable cushioning with a slightly sticky surface to prevent sliding. A yoga "sticky mat" is great for this too, but doesn't offer the same cushioning.

Stretch bands and resistance tubes The quality of bands is the same from reputable brands (*see Resources, p159*). Different-coloured bands denote different levels of resistance: light, medium, and heavy. Get at least two, either the light and medium, or the medium and heavy. The 1.2m (4ft) band length is more versatile than the 90cm (3ft). The rubber tubing comes with handles or foam pads, which may be easier to hold, if your hands are sensitive. You can also order handles for the bands.

Make sure that you store your equipment properly and check it periodically. The stretch bands should be powdered (with baby powder or cornflour) from time to time and stored flat in a plastic bag. You should untie them if you have knotted them up for an exercise. This will preserve the quality of their elasticity and prolong their life. In time the bands will deteriorate, become

tacky to touch, and may develop tiny holes and tears that can cause a break during use. This is the time to replace them.

Stability balls These generally come in 45-, 55-, 65- and 75-cm sizes; the size you use will depend on your height and the length of your legs. (Your knees should be bent at 90 degrees when you sit on the ball.) You will need a special ball pump to blow up your stability ball (a bicycle pump will not work).

Balls Weighted medicine balls offer options in all different sizes and weights. You might start with a 15–20cm (6–8in) unweighted ball (a beach ball is fine) and progress to a rubber or gel-filled medicine ball (1–6.7kg/2–15lb). I like to work with a 1.8kg (4lb) medicine ball because it offers good midlevel resistance.

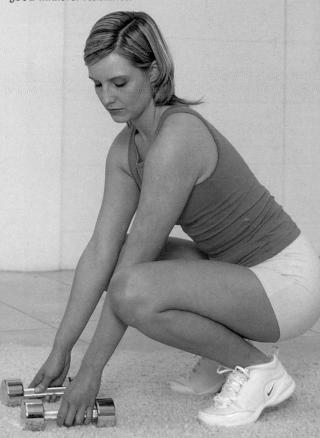

Correct form (*right*) Pick up free weights from the floor by bending your knees and keeping your spine straight; in this way your back is protected because the large muscles of the legs do the lifting.

POSTURE AND ALIGNMENT

Standing properly counteracts the constant force of gravity on the body, reducing stress on the spine and ensuring that the joints work efficiently. Muscles maintain the alignment of your skeletal frame when you are sitting, standing, or moving. Most of us have a natural tendency to muscular imbalance, with certain muscles being prone to shortening and others to lengthening and weakness. Resistance training combined with stretching can help correct these imbalances.

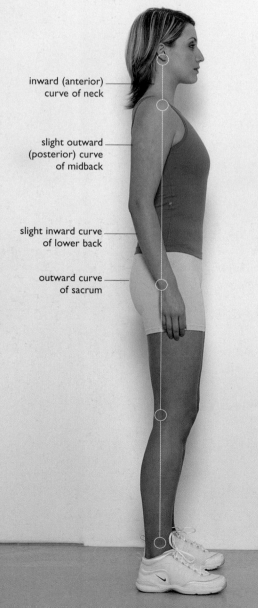

inward (anterior)
curve of neck

slight outward
(posterior) curve
of midback

slight inward curve
of lower back

outward curve
of sacrum

PROPER ALIGNMENT, SIDE VIEW:

What is good posture? The correct way to stand is with all the body's segments stacked from head to shoulders to hips, knees, and feet. An easy, reliable way to assess posture is to tie a length of string to something on the ceiling (a light fixture, for example) and put a light weight (such as a key ring) at the bottom of the string to weight it down. It forms a straight line. When you stand next to it sideways (*see left*), the centre of your ear, shoulder, hip, knee and ankle should be in a line. Do this with a partner to check each other out. The most common problems are forward head (with the chin jutting out), rounded shoulders, protruding abdomen, excessive curve in the lower back, and hyperextended knees.

Proper alignment for all standing exercises, front view
Stand in front of a mirror and check that your alignment is correct from the front:
• Stand with your feet parallel, hip-width apart. Feel your weight on the balls, outer edges, and heels of your feet; stand so you can lift up easily through the arches.
• Soften your knees so that they are not locked or hyperextended.
• Put your little fingers on your hipbones, and your thumbs on the bottom of your ribcage, and make sure your ribs are stacked on top of your hips, pelvis in neutral, i.e. not tilted forwards or backwards.
• Lift your chest; slide your shoulder blades down and together against the back of your ribcage.
• Centre your head right on top of the spinal column.

IMPROVING POSTURE

Poor posture can strain your joints and ultimately lead to headaches, neck and shoulder tension, sciatica, and hip and knee pain. Improving your posture can bring relief from all these conditions. In addition, as ancient meditation teachings stress, good posture is conducive to quieting the mind.

Good posture and poor posture are both habits that develop from repeated movement patterns. Get in the routine of doing a few simple exercises that will serve you for life.

Lengthening the spine To restore and maintain the normal curves of the spine, try this "growing exercise". Take a deep breath, filling the belly with air, and gradually lengthen the spine as you lift the top of your head to the ceiling. Think of elongating through the torso, stretching the space between the ribs and the hips, decompressing the spine. Fluff up the chest by drawing the air up into the chest cavity. As you exhale, hold the height and stay tall.

Realigning the pelvis The position of the pelvis determines the degree of curve in the lower back. Neutral lumbar spine alignment is midway between a full arch and a flat-back position (*see top right*). You should have a slight curve in the lower-back area, just enough to slip your hand in if you are lying on your back or standing straight with your back against the wall. If you have a flat back, stretch the hamstrings (*see p87*), since tight hamstrings pull the pelvis backwards. If you have a pronounced arch, or a hollow back, stretch the hip flexors in the front of the hip (*see p86*). Tight hip flexors pull the pelvis forwards.

Reversing a forward slouch The Neck Press (*see middle right*) works the muscles of the neck and upper back to bring the head back into alignment over the shoulder. The "Ws" (*see bottom right*) strengthen the muscles of the midback to keep it straight. Use your breath to create a rhythm for doing the exercises.

NEUTRAL SPINE ALIGNMENT

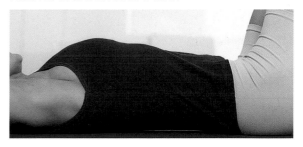

To get a good sense of neutral spine alignment, lie on your back with your knees bent. Do a strong pelvic tilt (*p50*), then release halfway, allowing the natural curve in the lower back.

NECK PRESS

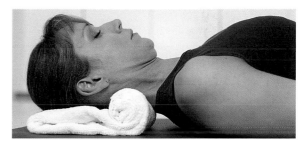

To strengthen the neck: lie on your back with your knees bent, feet flat on the floor. Put a small towel roll under your neck. Exhale on a count of 5 as you press the back of your neck into the towel (think of making a big double chin). Inhale as you release. Do 10 times daily.

"Ws" (ANCHORING THE SHOULDER BLADES)

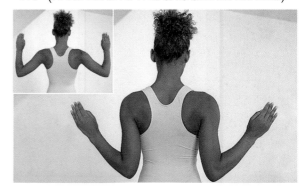

To strengthen the midback: hold your arms out to your sides, with the elbows bent to form a "W" (*top left*). Inhale, then squeeze the shoulder blades down and together as you slowly let your breath out. Repeat 10 times daily. Retraining comes through repetition.

CORE CONDITIONING

Once you are able to hold neutral spine alignment (*see pp24–25*) you are ready to move on to core conditioning. This combines strengthening, stretching, balance, and alignment training of the muscles that control the spine. Now you will challenge your abdominals and back muscles to work together as a team to stabilize the torso as you move. A strong core is the foundation for quality of movement in the whole body.

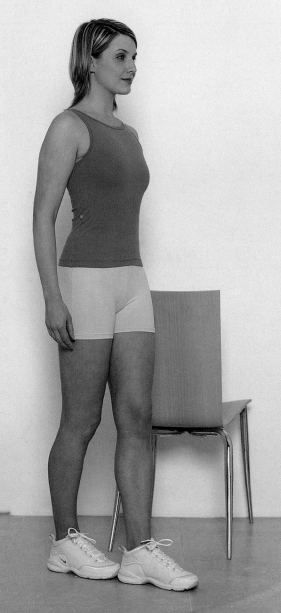

BALANCE TRAINING

An important aspect of core conditioning is balance training. With proper alignment, your weight-bearing joints are "stacked" for balance. Your balance centres — eyes, ears, and feet — work together to sense imbalance and correct posture. Your ability to balance peaks at around age 20 and normally remains excellent through early- to mid-40s. In the mid-40s, it begins a subtle process of deterioration, happening so slowly that it is almost imperceptible. Everyone has the ability to improve their balance, which reduces the risk of falling. Quicker reaction time, along with your ability to recover from a stumble or to change direction, can prevent an injury.

If you are just starting to work on balance, begin with the tandem stance (*see left*), which is a static position. To practise this, stand near a support (such as a sturdy chair) for safety, but try not to use it. Place one foot directly in front of the other, keeping your feet perfectly straight, and fix your eyes on something in front of you. When you can hold the position for 30 seconds, try closing your eyes (or one eye) to increase the level of difficulty.

Next, add movement for dynamic balance, such as walking in a straight line toe-to-heel or doing a lunge walk. Lunge forwards with one leg, bending both knees (*see pp69*), then step forwards with your back leg, bringing your feet together again. Lunge forwards with the other leg and repeat. Alternate lead feet, always bringing the feet together in between steps, so that you are travelling forwards as you lunge.

IMPROVING BALANCE

The next challenge to your equilibrium moves you from a stable surface, the floor, to an unstable one, the stability ball. You can sit, lie, or place your feet on top of the ball to create instability. Just sitting on it requires continual adjustments: the ball activates the muscles of your feet, legs, hips, and spine in order to maintain your balance. Some schools in Europe have replaced chairs with balls in classrooms to improve posture and activity levels in children. I use one myself for a desk chair.

The ball is also an excellent tool for improving co-ordination. One of the best ways to correct faulty movement patterns is to work on an unstable base of support, where ingrained habits can no longer dominate. Motor relearning occurs when newly organized movement patterns emerge from the "chaos" you initially feel.

The correct ball size is based on your height and the length of your legs — when you sit on the ball, your hips and knees should be bent at 90-degree angles. Using the wrong size ball can be uncomfortable and even harmful to the spine and the joints.

The easiest way to start working on a stability ball is to lie on the floor on your back, with your lower legs resting on the ball, knees bent at 90 degrees (*see Ball Bridge, pp77*). To work in a tabletop or prone position on the ball, it is important to get into position and to come off the ball safely. Follow the guidelines at the right.

FUNCTIONAL TRAINING

Integrating all these aspects of training prepares your whole body to meet the demands of your day-to-day activities more effectively (i.e. functional training). You'll appreciate it the next time you are walking home on a wet, windy day, holding an open umbrella in one hand, a tote bag slung over the opposite shoulder, and carrying several shopping bags in the other hand, and you want to buy a newspaper without falling over. This is the pay off of functional training. Working on the stability ball in particular is a good tool for functional training.

TABLETOP POSITION

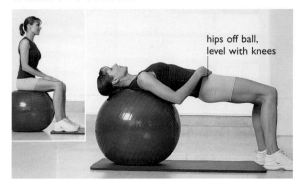

hips off ball, level with knees

Sit on the ball with your knees bent at 90 degrees. If you are just learning, hold onto the sides of the ball as you walk your feet forwards and slide down until your head, neck, and shoulders are supported. To return to an upright position, walk your feet in towards the ball as you curl forwards.

PRONE POSITION

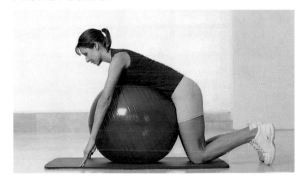

1 Kneel on the mat, face down over the ball so that your torso is on top of the ball. Roll forwards a little until only your fingers, knees, and toes are on the floor.

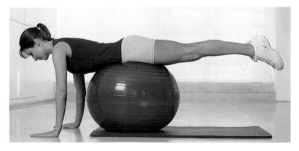

2 Slowly walk the body away from the ball with the hands, until your hips (or knees) are resting on the ball, hands planted on the floor. To come off, reverse the movement.

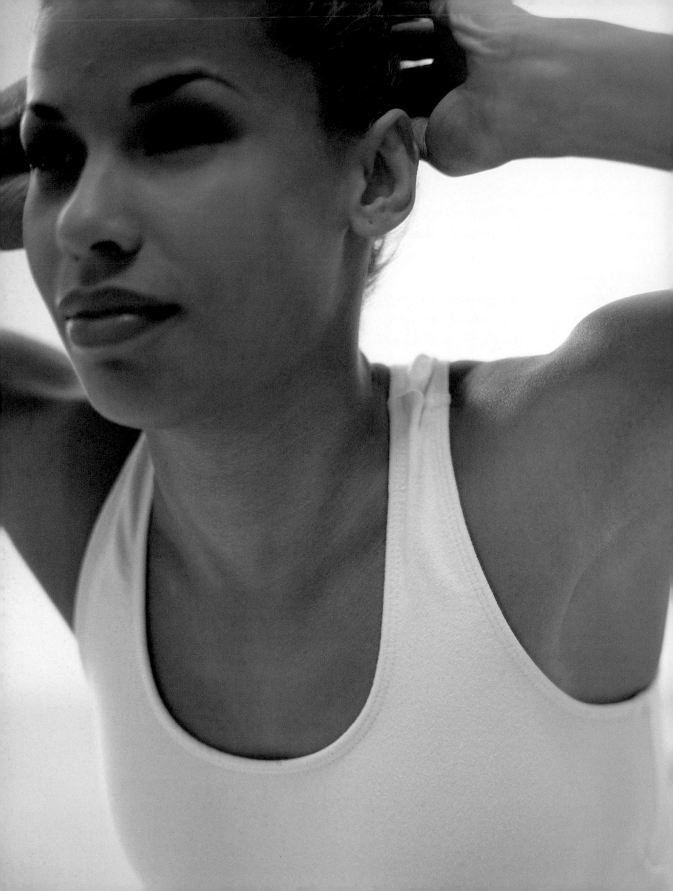

4 FOR LIFE

We start our resistance-training programme with four simple

exercises – a squat, a press-up, a back extension, and a pelvic

tilt. Together, they provide a mini full-body conditioning workout

that uses body weight only and that you can do almost

anywhere, any time. Even if you never go on to the rest of the

exercises in this book, your body will benefit enormously from

doing these four moves regularly. Use them as the building

blocks of your programme and the baseline to which you

return if you are short of time. When life becomes hectic,

they are the ideal "active rest" from your full programme.

"I started working out with Joan in my mid-40s primarily out of a desire
not to end up like my mother, who has health issues related to smoking
and lack of exercise. As my muscles toned up, a whole new shape emerged.
I look younger and I feel more energized and in control." *Jean R-M.*

PROGRAMMES AT A GLANCE

If you are new to exercise, or if you are very out of shape, you should start with the Level 1 programme below. Do the exercises at least twice a week, and add the band exercises to strengthen key postural muscles when you have time. When you are ready, you can either progress to the next levels or move on to the programmes in the rest of the book.

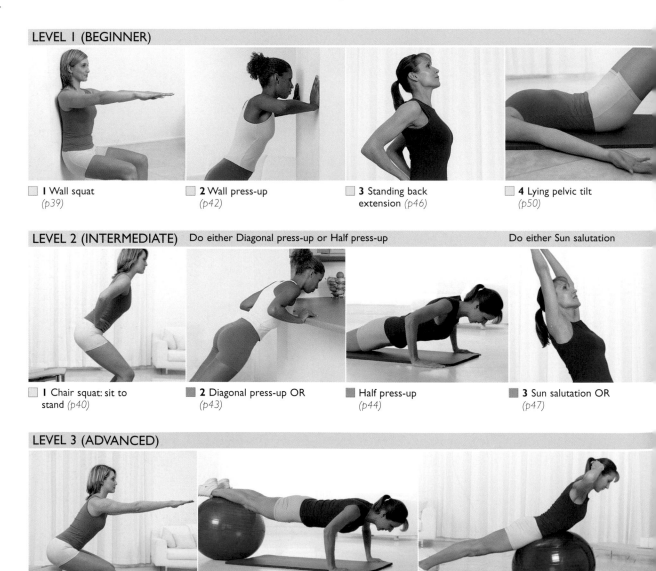

LEVEL 1 (BEGINNER)

☐ **1** Wall squat *(p39)*

☐ **2** Wall press-up *(p42)*

☐ **3** Standing back extension *(p46)*

☐ **4** Lying pelvic tilt *(p50)*

LEVEL 2 (INTERMEDIATE)   Do either Diagonal press-up or Half press-up   Do either Sun salutation

☐ **1** Chair squat: sit to stand *(p40)*

■ **2** Diagonal press-up OR *(p43)*

■ Half press-up *(p44)*

■ **3** Sun salutation OR *(p47)*

LEVEL 3 (ADVANCED)

■ **1** Chair squat: stand to sit *(p41)*

■ **2** Full press-up on ball *(p45)*

■ **3** Back extension on ball *(p49)*

TRAINING GUIDELINES

- Remember to warm up (*pp32–37*) before you start and to stretch out (*pp54–55*) after working the muscles.
- Use proper body alignment and good form.
- Start gently and avoid pain.
- Gradually increase the intensity.

- Use the colour code to guide you in your choice of exercise:

  Beginner: suitable for most people

  Intermediate: requires more strength and coordination

  Advanced: challenges strength and balance

Posture Plus

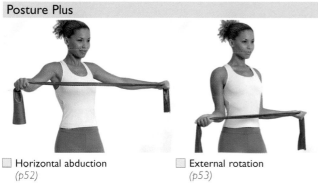

☐ Horizontal abduction (*p52*) ☐ External rotation (*p53*)

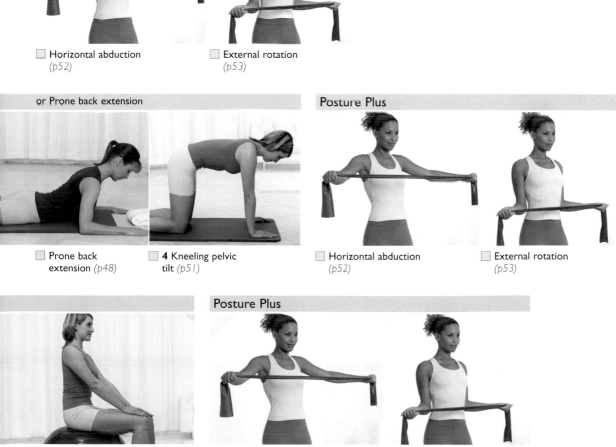

or Prone back extension

☐ Prone back extension (*p48*) ☐ **4** Kneeling pelvic tilt (*p51*)

Posture Plus

☐ Horizontal abduction (*p52*) ☐ External rotation (*p53*)

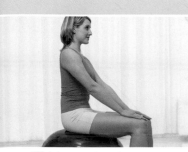

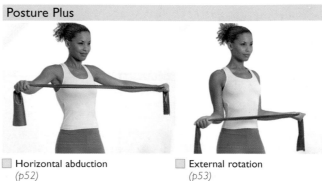

■ **4** Sitting pelvic tilt (*p51*)

Posture Plus

☐ Horizontal abduction (*p52*) ☐ External rotation (*p53*)

WARMING UP

The warm-up prepares the body for more strenuous work and reduces the risk of injury. Performing any series of rhythmic movements for 5 minutes or so will increase blood flow to your muscles, making them warm and pliable, and lubricate the joints. Repeat the ball series 2 or 3 times until you feel warm and break a light sweat. The pre-stretches with the band (*pp35–37*) work the range of motion in the shoulder joint and lengthen the muscles throughout the body.

☐ BODY-BALL REACH

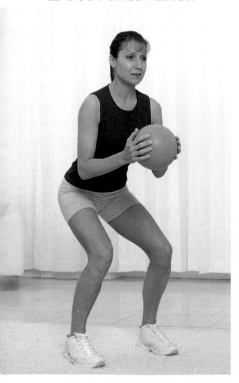

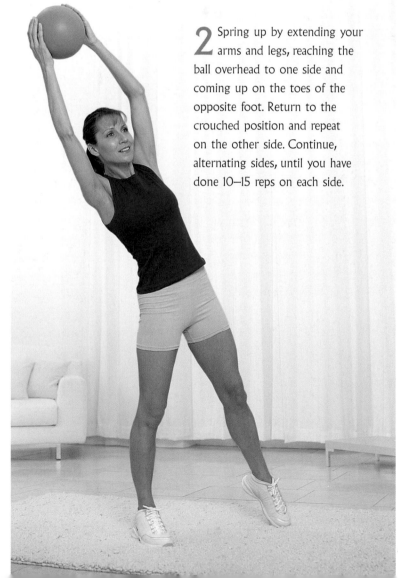

2 Spring up by extending your arms and legs, reaching the ball overhead to one side and coming up on the toes of the opposite foot. Return to the crouched position and repeat on the other side. Continue, alternating sides, until you have done 10–15 reps on each side.

1 Stand with your knees bent in a crouched position, feet parallel and hip-width apart. Hold a 19-cm (7½-in) ball close to your body with your arms bent. (If you want to make the ball exercises more strenuous, use a weighted ball.)

☐ KNEE LIFT WITH BALL

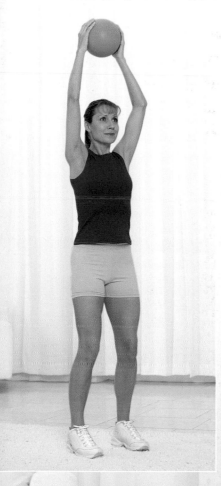

TRAINER'S TIPS

● **Your weight** should be centred over the arches of your feet, not leaning forwards over your toes or backwards onto your heels.
● **Keep your arches** lifted so that your feet do not roll inwards or outwards.
● **Lift your chest** and look straight ahead.

2 Lower the ball to chest height and at the same time bring one knee up to touch it. Return to the start position and switch legs. Repeat, alternating sides, until you have done 10–15 reps on each side.

1 Stand with your feet parallel, hip-width apart, knees soft. Tighten your abdominals to stabilize your torso. Hold the ball overhead with both hands.

☐ PLIÉ WITH BALL LIFT

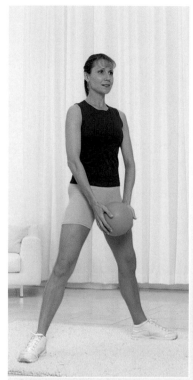

2 Inhale as you bend your knees and lift the ball to chest height. Think "bend and lift". Exhale as you straighten your legs and lower the ball to return to the start position, pressing through your heels and squeezing your inner thighs and buttocks as you come up. Repeat 10–15 times.

1 Stand with your legs slightly wider than hip-width apart. Shift your weight to the heels and turn the legs and feet out from the hip as a unit until the feet are at 45-degrees. Hold the ball down in front of you.

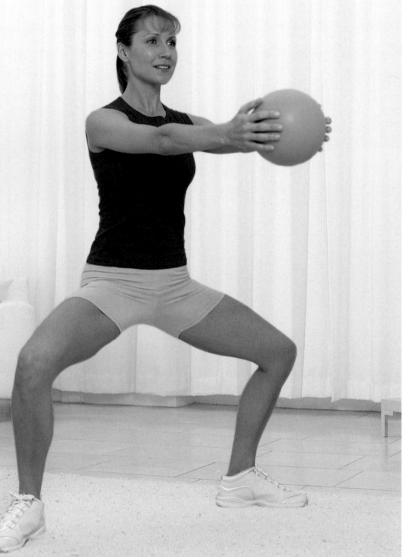

■ SHOULDER ROTATION

This stretch lengthens the muscles and connective tissue around the shoulder joint. Use a light to medium band.

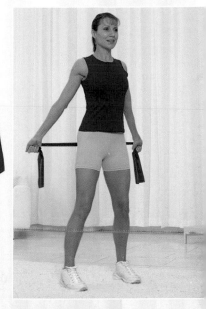

1 Put a little tension in the band and hold it in front of you at shoulder height, arms wide. Your palms are facing down, wrists flat. Slowly reach your arms overhead. You will feel a pull in the front of the shoulders. If the pull is too intense, move your hands farther apart to get a wider grip on the band, or use the bent-arm position (*see box, right*).

2 Use caution as you lower the band behind you, all the way down to your hips, keeping your elbows straight. Reverse the movement to return the band to the start position. Repeat the whole movement 8 times.

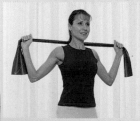

BENT ARMS
If this stretch is new to you, start with your elbows bent in front of you. Do not reach up high, just take the band to the back of your shoulders in Step 2.

SIDE-BEND STRETCH

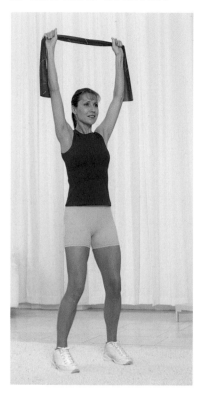

1 Stand with your feet parallel, hip-width apart, knees soft. Put a little tension in the band and hold it overhead, palms facing forwards. Reach for the sky, with your arms slightly wider than shoulder-width apart. Keep your shoulder blades anchored and your wrists flat. Centre your head between your elbows.

2 Still reaching for the sky, flex to the side at the waist, then return to centre and flex to the other side. Repeat, alternating sides, until you have done 8 reps on each side, always stopping at centre as you switch sides.

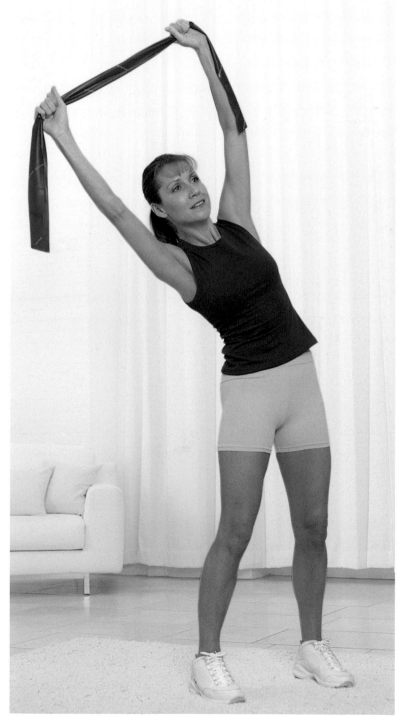

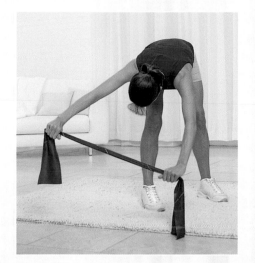

SIDE BEND WITH TWIST

This is a great full-body stretch if you do not have lower back pain or a spinal condition. Move straight from your last side bend to this exercise.

1 Take a side bend to the right (*see Step 2, opposite*) and, maintaining tension in the band, bend forwards from the waist and circle your torso towards the floor.

2 Continue to circle to come up on your left side, twisting your torso back to centre as you stand up. Your right arm leads as you come up out of the circle and return to the start position. Reverse direction and repeat, alternating sides, until you have done 8 reps on each side.

TRAINER'S TIPS

- **Plant your feet** securely, but keep your knees bent softly.
- **Maintain tension** in the band throughout.
- **Your head** should be centred between your elbows.
- **Keep your shoulder blades** drawn down to anchor them.

1 SQUATS

If I were to give everyone one exercise for life, the squat would be it. By working the muscles of the thighs, the buttocks, and the lower legs, as well as using the abdominal and back muscles to stabilize the torso, the squat is the closest we can get to a full-body exercise. It is the same movement that we need to rise from a seated position, or to bend down to the floor, so it is a very functional exercise that helps to keep us independent as we advance in years. To reduce stress on the knees, master the proper form; in particular, make sure you keep your weight back on your heels.

KEY MUSCLES INVOLVED

Gluteals

Quadriceps

Hamstring group

Iliotibial band

Hamstring group

Squats work all the major muscle groups in the upper part of the leg: the buttocks (gluteals) and the thighs (quadriceps and hamstrings).

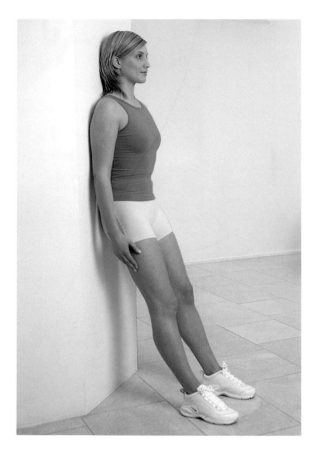

WALL SQUAT

To strengthen your knees, begin with the Wall Squat, in which you lean some of your body weight against the wall and slide up and down. This exercise is also called the Olympic Rest because it is a great ski-conditioning exercise that can be done outdoors, leaning against a tree. For this kind of endurance training, hold the position for as long as you can (up to 90 seconds).

1 Stand with your back against the wall. Take a giant step out and plant both feet securely on the floor. Your feet should be parallel, hip-width apart. Keep your head, shoulders, and buttocks pressed into the wall. Draw in your abdominals.

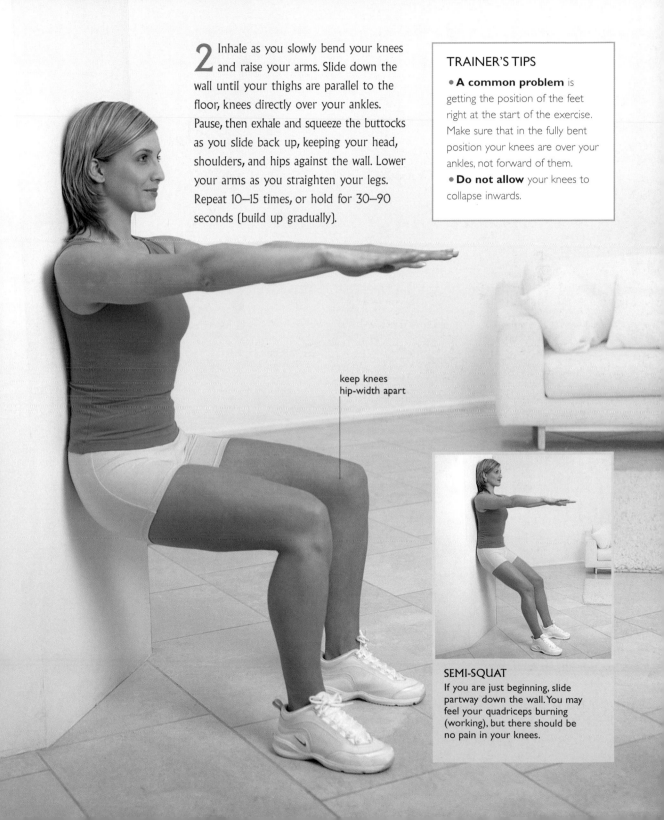

2 Inhale as you slowly bend your knees and raise your arms. Slide down the wall until your thighs are parallel to the floor, knees directly over your ankles. Pause, then exhale and squeeze the buttocks as you slide back up, keeping your head, shoulders, and hips against the wall. Lower your arms as you straighten your legs. Repeat 10–15 times, or hold for 30–90 seconds (build up gradually).

TRAINER'S TIPS

- **A common problem** is getting the position of the feet right at the start of the exercise. Make sure that in the fully bent position your knees are over your ankles, not forward of them.
- **Do not allow** your knees to collapse inwards.

keep knees
hip-width apart

SEMI-SQUAT
If you are just beginning, slide partway down the wall. You may feel your quadriceps burning (working), but there should be no pain in your knees.

☐ CHAIR SQUAT: SIT TO STAND

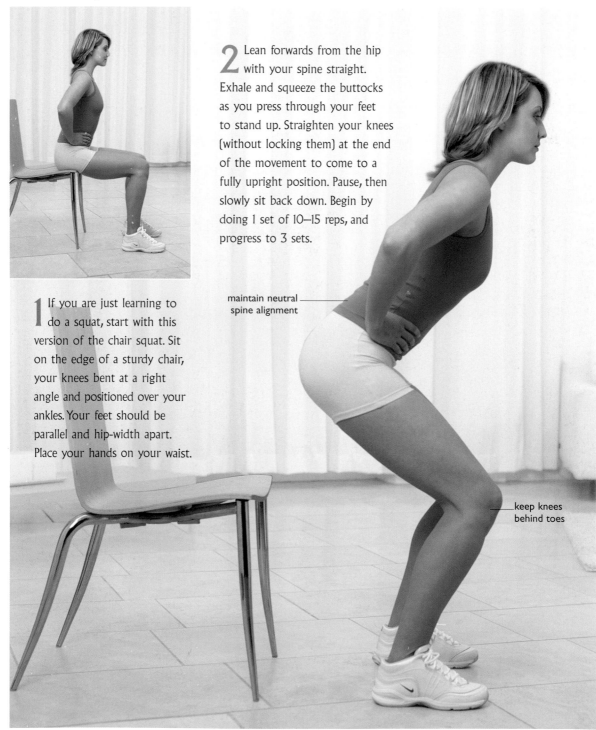

2 Lean forwards from the hip with your spine straight. Exhale and squeeze the buttocks as you press through your feet to stand up. Straighten your knees (without locking them) at the end of the movement to come to a fully upright position. Pause, then slowly sit back down. Begin by doing 1 set of 10–15 reps, and progress to 3 sets.

1 If you are just learning to do a squat, start with this version of the chair squat. Sit on the edge of a sturdy chair, your knees bent at a right angle and positioned over your ankles. Your feet should be parallel and hip-width apart. Place your hands on your waist.

maintain neutral spine alignment

keep knees behind toes

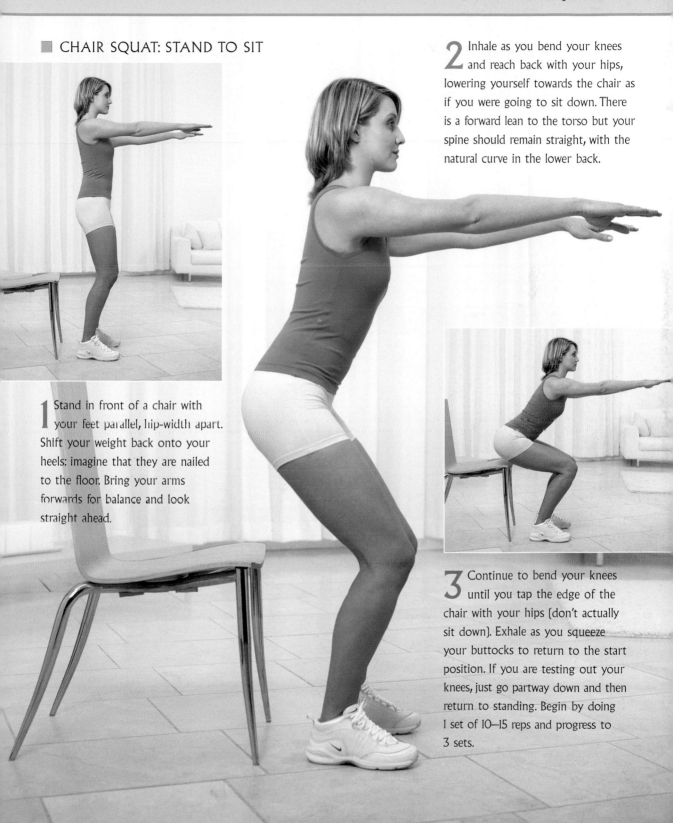

■ CHAIR SQUAT: STAND TO SIT

1 Stand in front of a chair with your feet parallel, hip-width apart. Shift your weight back onto your heels: imagine that they are nailed to the floor. Bring your arms forwards for balance and look straight ahead.

2 Inhale as you bend your knees and reach back with your hips, lowering yourself towards the chair as if you were going to sit down. There is a forward lean to the torso but your spine should remain straight, with the natural curve in the lower back.

3 Continue to bend your knees until you tap the edge of the chair with your hips (don't actually sit down). Exhale as you squeeze your buttocks to return to the start position. If you are testing out your knees, just go partway down and then return to standing. Begin by doing 1 set of 10–15 reps and progress to 3 sets.

② PRESS-UPS

The press-up uses body weight to work multiple muscles in an integrated way – in the same way that your body moves in daily life. While the pectorals, deltoid, and triceps are all involved in the movement, the position of your hands determines which muscle you emphasize: wide for the chest, narrow for the shoulders. All press-ups help firm the triceps in the back of the arm and are weight-bearing through the arms and the wrists. The abdominals and back muscles are active in stabilizing the torso. The level of difficulty is determined by how much weight you shift onto your upper body.

KEY MUSCLES INVOLVED

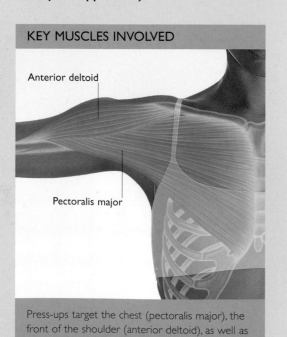

Anterior deltoid

Pectoralis major

Press-ups target the chest (pectoralis major), the front of the shoulder (anterior deltoid), as well as the back of the arm (triceps).

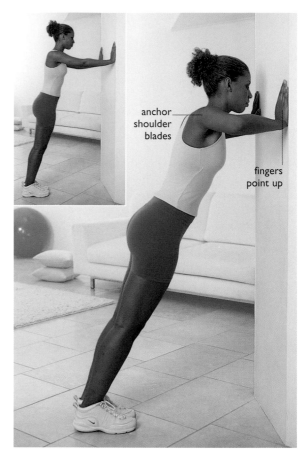

anchor shoulder blades

fingers point up

☐ WALL PRESS-UP

I encourage my clients to find an unobstructed wall in their homes that will be their "press-up station" and every time they pass that wall, to do a few reps. It is the least demanding version of the press-up because you are lifting the least body weight. The wide position of the hands targets the chest.

Stand a full arms' length away from the wall, your hands at shoulder level, but 7.5–10cm (3–4in) wider than your shoulders. Pull your abdominals in tight so that there is a straight line from your shoulders to your ankles. Inhale and bend your elbows out to the sides to 90 degrees as you lower your chest towards the wall. Exhale and push back to the start position. Repeat 10–15 times.

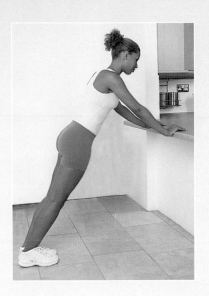

■ DIAGONAL PRESS-UP

This version of the press-up is harder because you shift more body weight onto your upper body as you lower into a diagonal position. Keeping your elbows in close to your sides targets the deltoid. Be sure to use a fixed support, such as a kitchen counter or a ballet barre.

1 Stand an arms' length away from the support with your arms straight, your hands shoulder-width apart, fingers pointing straight ahead. Draw your shoulder blades down and together. Pull your abdominals in tight so that your body is in a straight line.

2 Inhale and bend your elbows in close to your sides as you lower your chest to the counter. Allow your heels to roll off the floor. (For additional resistance, stay up on your toes throughout the entire exercise to shift more body weight onto your upper body). Exhale and push back to the start position. Repeat 10–15 times.

TRAINER'S TIPS

- **Anchor your shoulder** blades by drawing them down and together before you move.
- **Keep your head** and neck aligned with your spine.
- **Pull your abdominals** tight to stop the lower back from sagging.
- **Your arms** should be straight but not stiff when extended.

■ HALF PRESS-UP

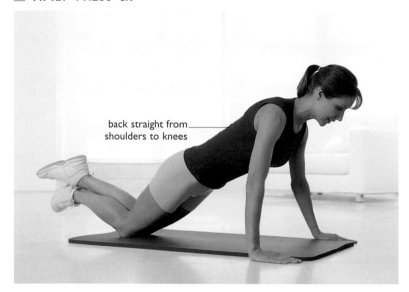

back straight from shoulders to knees

If you have problems with your wrists, stick with the Wall Press-Up on p42, since this will cause less stress to them.

1 Kneel on the mat with your wrists in line with your shoulders but 7.5–10cm (3–4in) wider than shoulder-width apart. Your fingers should point forwards. Drop your hips and shift your weight forwards onto your arms so that there is no direct pressure on your kneecaps. Cross your ankles and relax your lower legs.

2 Anchor your shoulder blades by drawing them down and together. Inhale and bend your elbows out to the sides to form a box as you slowly lower your chest towards the floor. Exhale as you straighten your arms and push up to the start position. Begin with 1 set of 15–20 reps and build up to 2 sets.

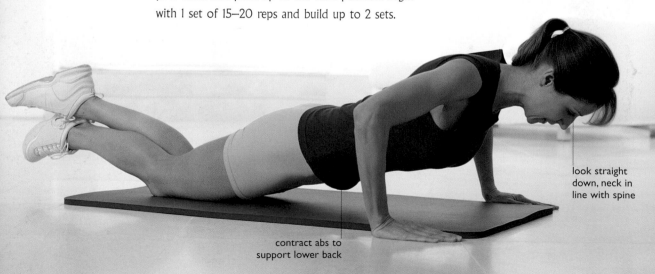

look straight down, neck in line with spine

contract abs to support lower back

■ FULL PRESS-UP ON BALL

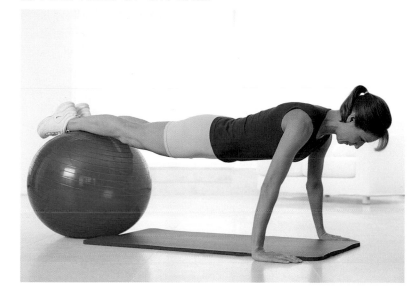

This exercise may look dramatic, but it is easier to do than a full press-up on the floor because you can regulate how much body weight you shift onto your arms. The farther you walk out on the stability ball, the more you load your upper body.

1 Lengthen out over the ball as far as you can, while staying stable and in control of the weight on your arms. The hands should be in line with the shoulders, but slightly wider than shoulder-width apart.

2 Anchor your shoulder blades. Inhale and bend your elbows out to the sides as you slowly lower your chest towards the floor. Exhale as you straighten your arms and push up to the start position. To begin, do 1 set of 15–20 reps and work up to 2 sets.

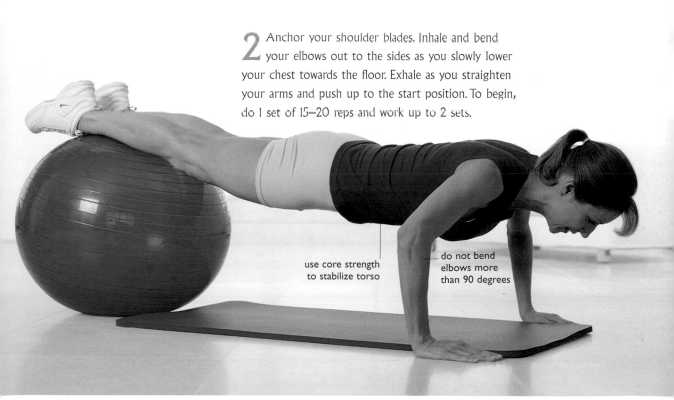

use core strength to stabilize torso

do not bend elbows more than 90 degrees

③ BACK EXTENSIONS

To maintain a youthful appearance, forget the fancy rejuvenating creams and try back extensions instead. My strategy costs far less and delivers more dramatic results. Back extensions trigger the erector spinae group, strengthening the muscles that run the length of your spine so that you stand taller and straighter. They also improve mobility in the upper and middle back. As you lift your chest and arch your upper back, you open the front of the shoulders to create a young, confident posture.

KEY MUSCLES INVOLVED

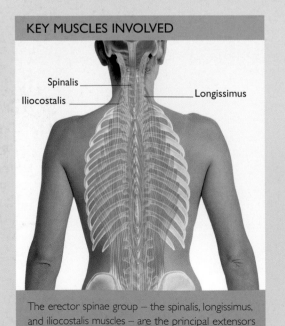

Spinalis

Iliocostalis

Longissimus

The erector spinae group – the spinalis, longissimus, and iliocostalis muscles – are the principal extensors of the spine.

☐ STANDING BACK EXTENSION

If you are not used to bending backwards, begin with this version. To avoid any compression in the lower back, lengthen through the spine by lifting the top of the head towards the ceiling before you start to arch.

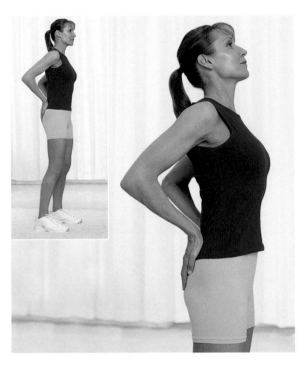

Stand with your feet parallel, hip-width apart, knees soft. Place your hands on your buttocks below your waist. Take a deep breath and lengthen the torso. Exhale and lift the chest up as you pull your elbows towards each other, causing the upper back to arch slightly. Release back to centre and repeat 5–10 times.

WORKING UP THE SPINE

As you increase your mobility, move your hands up the back in stages. Make two fists, plant them close together on the back of the waist, and perform the exercise. When you are ready to progress, move the fists higher up, above the waist.

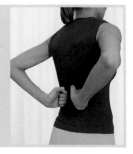

■ SUN SALUTATION

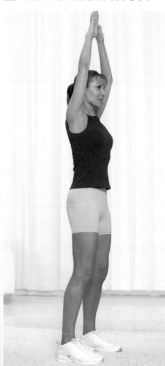

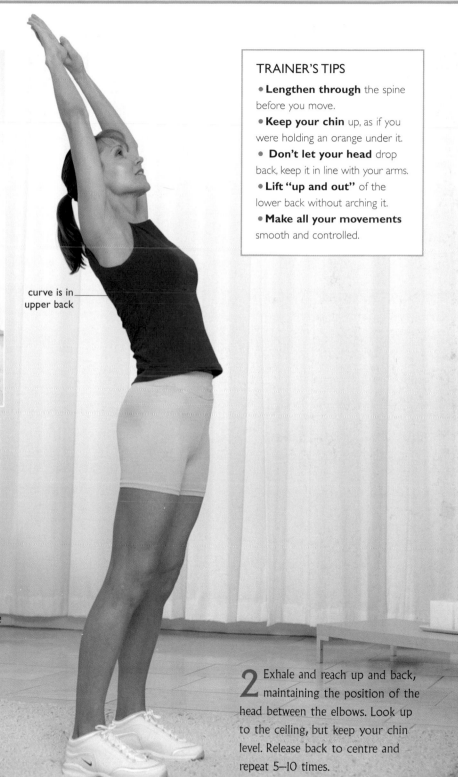

curve is in upper back

This is a wonderful full-body stretch to counteract tight, shortened muscles. My 92-year-old client loves this movement.

1 Stand with your feet parallel, hip-width apart. Interlock your thumbs and reach your arms overhead, keeping your head between your elbows. Inhale, and lengthen through the spine. Tighten your hips, thighs, and buttocks to protect your lower back.

2 Exhale and reach up and back, maintaining the position of the head between the elbows. Look up to the ceiling, but keep your chin level. Release back to centre and repeat 5–10 times.

☐ PRONE BACK EXTENSION

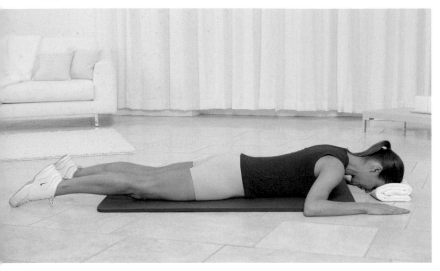

Attempt this exercise only if your lower back is free of pain. The only sensation you should feel while performing it is the muscles of the lower back tightening as they work.

1 Lie face down on the mat with a folded towel under your forehead to ensure proper alignment of the head and neck with the spine. Bend your arms and rest your forearms on the floor, palms down. Scoop out the abdomen to support the lower back.

TRAINER'S TIPS

• **Contract your abdominals** by drawing your belly button towards the spine.

• **If your lower back** arches excessively, use a folded towel under the pelvis (or hips) to even out the spinal alignment.

• **Keep your hips** pressed into the floor.

2 Lengthen the spine by reaching forwards with the top of the head. Draw your shoulder blades down and together. Exhale as you lift your head and shoulders off the floor; do not use any strength from your arms. Keep your nose down. Pause at the top, then inhale and slowly return to the start position without resting. Begin with 10 reps and build up to 1 set of 15–20 reps.

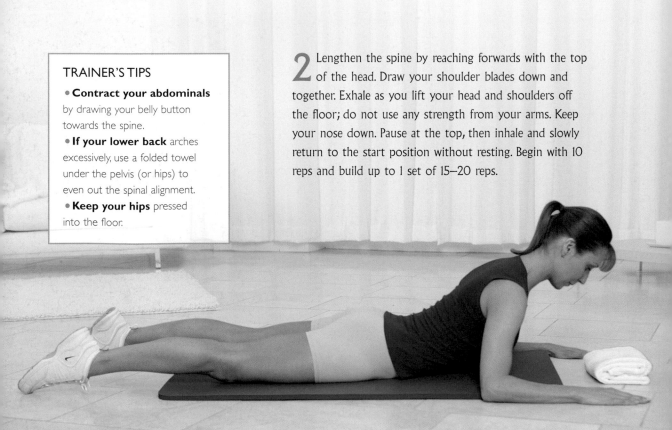

■ BACK EXTENSION ON BALL

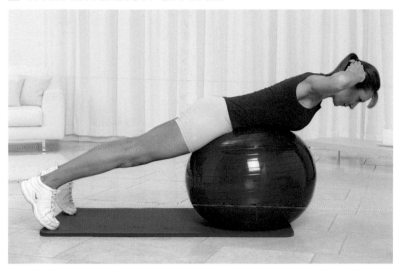

This advanced version requires you to stabilize the full length of your body while challenging you with increased resistance (hands behind your head) and greater range of motion (more height to the lift).

1 Position your torso on the stability ball with your legs extended and dig your toes into the mat. Alternatively, plant your feet against a wall. Rest your fingertips lightly at the back of your head and lengthen your spine.

2 Exhale as you squeeze your buttocks and slowly lift your torso to 15 degrees. Press your hips into the ball. Pause at the top, then inhale and slowly return to the start position without resting. Begin with 10 reps and build up to 1 set of 15–20 reps.

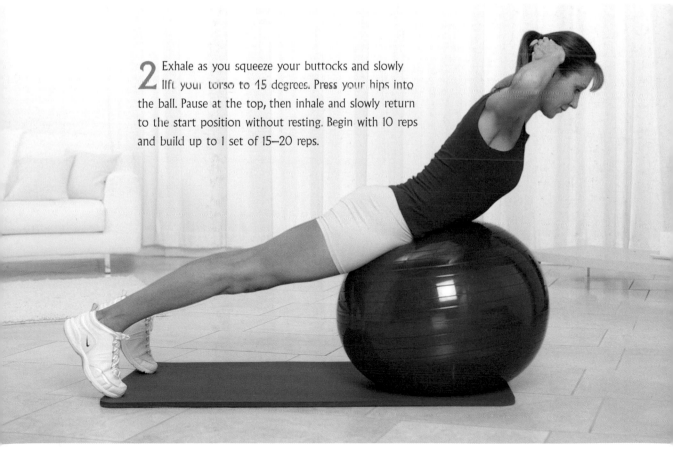

4 PELVIC TILTS

The basis for all abdominal work is diaphragmatic breathing. Although it is intuitive to all of us, most of us breathe shallowly from the chest in our upright posture and we need to relearn it. Watch a baby breathe and you will see that the abdomen expands on the inhale and contracts on the exhale. The pelvic tilt combines this breathing pattern with abdominal compression and a slight rotation of the hips, strengthening the abdomen and stretching the lower back.

KEY MUSCLES INVOLVED

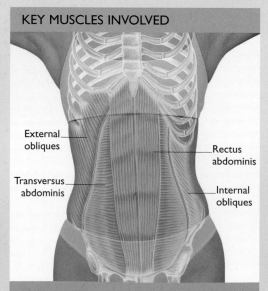

External obliques

Rectus abdominis

Transversus abdominis

Internal obliques

Pelvic tilts work the four major muscles of the abdomen – the transversus abdominis, the rectus abdominis, and the internal and external obliques – and stretch the erector spinae.

☐ LYING PELVIC TILT

Although pelvic tilts can be done properly in many positions, start with the easiest – lying flat on your back – while you practise coordinating the breath with the abdominal action.

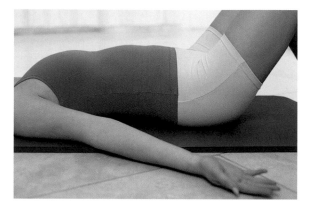

1 Lie on your back on the mat with your knees bent, feet flat on the floor. Rest your arms by your sides, palms up. Your spine should be in neutral, with the natural curve in the lower back. Inhale and bring the breath into the abdomen, filling the belly with air.

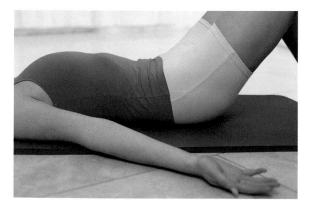

2 Exhale forcefully by pulling your abdominals in tight – think "belly button to spine" – pushing the air out. With one fluid motion, flatten your lower back into the floor and curl your hips 2.5cm (1in) off the floor. Release back to the start position and repeat 10–15 times.

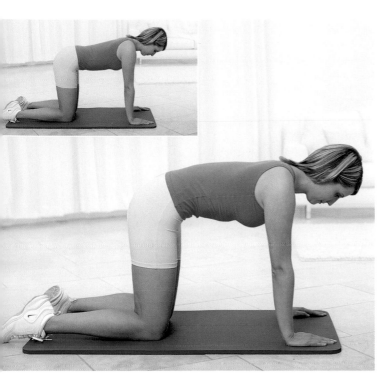

☐ KNEELING PELVIC TILT

This position is helpful for anyone who is not able to lie flat. Some experts recommend avoiding the supine position on the opposite page after the first trimester of pregnancy because it may interfere with blood supply to the fetus.

Kneel on the mat with your hands under your shoulders and your knees under your hips, your back in neutral spine alignment. Inhale, filling the belly with air. Exhale forcefully, pulling your abdominals in tight, drawing the belly button towards the spine. With one fluid motion, reverse the curve in the lower back and tilt your hips under. Release and repeat 10–15 times.

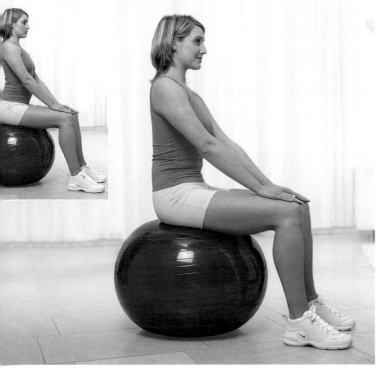

■ SITTING PELVIC TILT

It is more difficult to perform the pelvic tilt in an upright posture, standing or sitting, but doing this exercise on a stability ball provides a helpful cue, as the ball will shift forwards slightly when you do the movement correctly.

Sit up tall on the ball, your feet parallel, hip-width apart. Rest your hands on your knees. Keep your back straight, in neutral spine alignment. Inhale and fill your belly with air. Exhale forcefully, pulling your abdominals in tight, drawing the belly button towards the spine. With one fluid motion, reverse the curve in the lower back by tucking your hips under, rolling the ball forwards 2.5cm (1in). Release and repeat 10–15 times.

POSTURE PLUS

Add a stretch band to target key muscles of the shoulder and upper back. Whenever someone compliments me on my posture, I share this secret with them: two powerful exercises to counteract slouching. Horizontal abduction strengthens the midback muscles (rhomboids and midtrapezius) and, together with external rotation, the back of the shoulder (posterior deltoid and external rotators).

WEIGHTS & REPETITIONS

Shaping and toning Light to medium band. Do 12–15 reps per set.

Bone building Heavy band. Do 8–12 reps per set.

◻ HORIZONTAL ABDUCTION

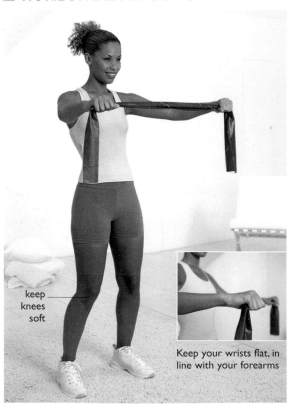

keep knees soft

Keep your wrists flat, in line with your forearms

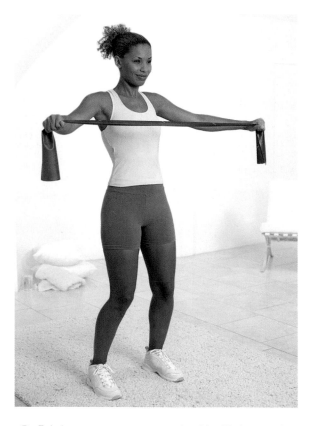

1 Stand with your feet parallel, hip-width apart. Hold the band at chest height with your palms down, your arms slightly wider than shoulder-width apart. Your elbows should be rounded; your wrists flat. Anchor the shoulder blades and put a little tension in the band.

2 Exhale as you squeeze your shoulder blades together and pull the band into your chest. Keep your elbows rounded at a constant angle and pull from the back of your shoulders. Pause briefly, then inhale as you slowly release back to the start position.

■ EXTERNAL ROTATION

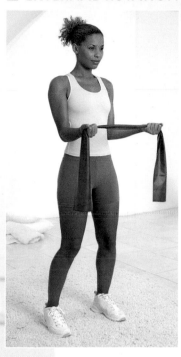

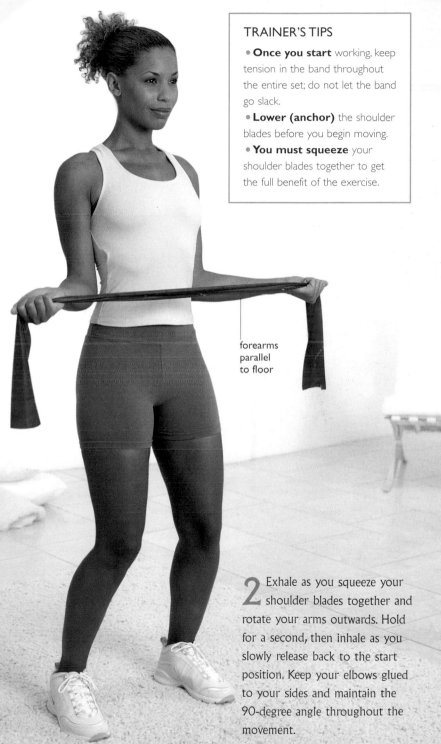

forearms parallel to floor

1 Stand with your feet parallel, hip-width apart, knees soft. Hold the band with your palms up, elbows bent at a right angle and close to your sides. Anchor your shoulder blades and put a little tension in the band.

2 Exhale as you squeeze your shoulder blades together and rotate your arms outwards. Hold for a second, then inhale as you slowly release back to the start position. Keep your elbows glued to your sides and maintain the 90-degree angle throughout the movement.

COOLING DOWN STRETCHES

After you have worked your muscles, it is important to stretch them out to lengthen them and to release tension. Regular stretching makes you taller, more agile, and even stronger – it can increase strength gains by up to 20 per cent. Breathe into the stretch as you hold each position for 10–15 seconds. Breathe naturally during the shoulder rolls.

☐ CHEST STRETCH

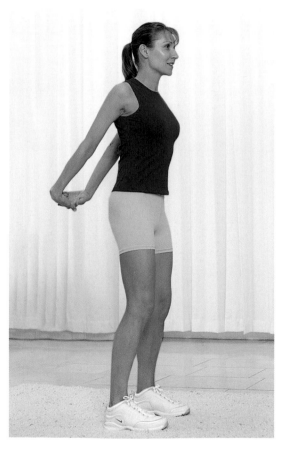

Stand with your feet parallel, hip-width apart, knees soft. Clasp your hands behind your back and raise them towards the ceiling as you lift your chest. Keep your chin level and look straight ahead.

☐ UPPER-BACK STRETCH

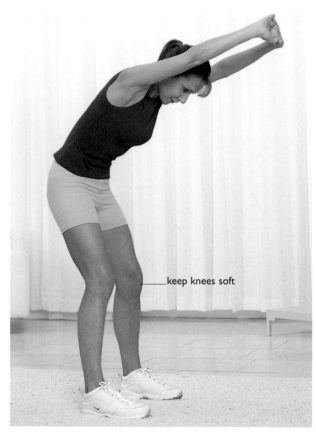

keep knees soft

Stand with your feet parallel, hip-width apart, knees soft. Clasp your hands overhead and turn your palms to the ceiling. Reach forwards as you round the upper back. Keep your head between your elbows.

☐ LAT STRETCH

☐ TORSO STRETCH

☐ SHOULDER ROLLS

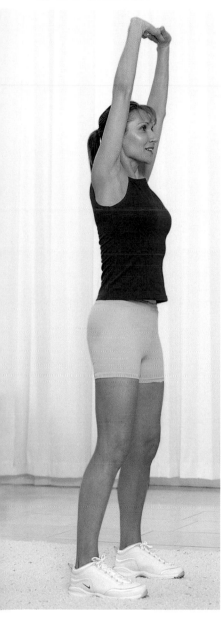

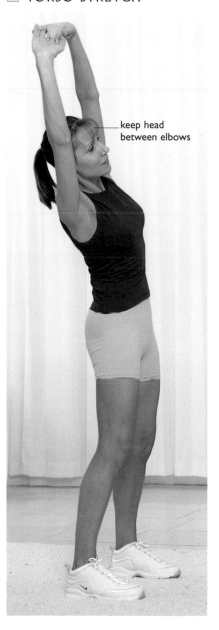

keep head between elbows

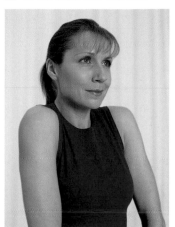

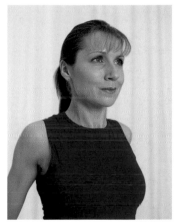

Initiate the movement from the shoulder blades. First, shrug the shoulders, then roll them back and together. To reverse the circle, separate the shoulder blades to bring the shoulders forwards. Repeat 3 times each way.

Stand with your feet parallel, hip-width apart, knees soft. Clasp your hands overhead and turn your palms to the ceiling. Reach for the sky, lengthening through the torso. Feel the stretch along your back.

From the previous position, imagine your body is between two plates of glass. Maintain that alignment, and reach your arms to one side and then the other, feeling a stretch all the way down to your hips.

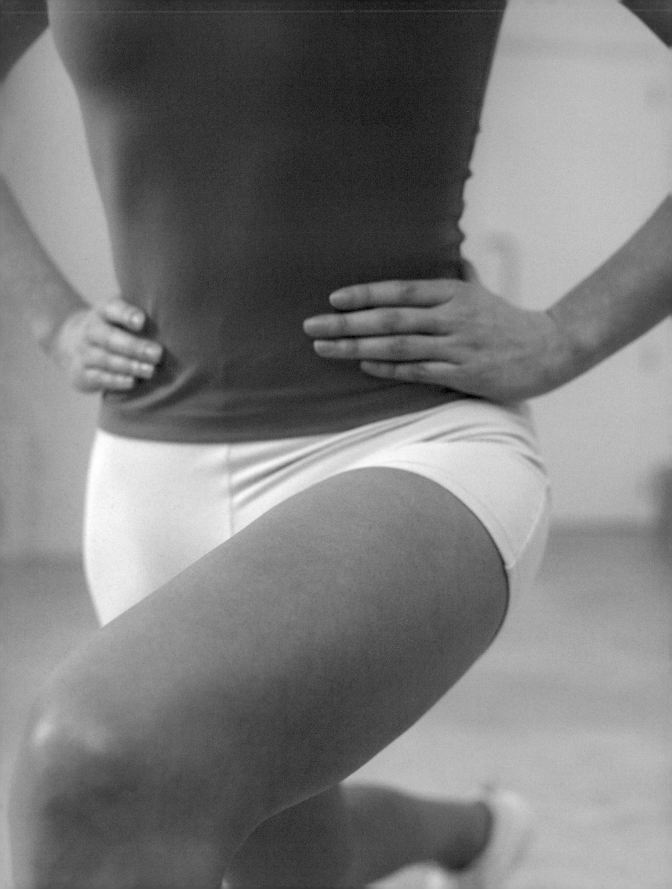

LOWER BODY PROGRAMME

We begin our full weight-training programme with the hips and thighs, since these comprise the largest muscle group of the body. The following exercises will keep you lean in your jeans, lifting the buttocks, firming the thighs, and sculpting the calves. Shaping the lower body can be a powerful motivation, but these exercises also strengthen the large muscles of the legs that keep us active, stable, and self-sufficient as we age. To get the most out of your programme, vary your lower-body exercises from time to time, picking different tools, such as the weights, tubes, and stability ball.

"Joan's passion has kept me energized throughout more than 15 years of working out, despite my utter hatred of exercise. It is truly a testament to how wonderful she is!" *Josie N.*

PROGRAMMES AT A GLANCE

Work through the programmes below, starting with Level 1 and building up to Level 3. Alternatively, create your own whole-body programme of 8–10 exercises, starting with three exercises to target the glutes and thighs and one for the calves. Be sure to master the proper form of the squat (*pp38–41*) before adding the challenge of weights and tubes.

LEVEL 1 (BEGINNER)

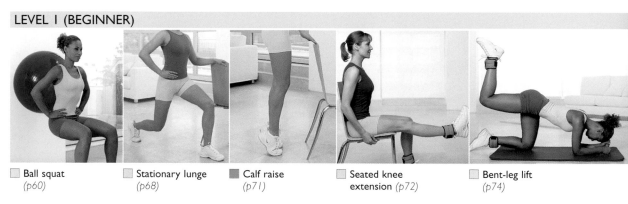

☐ Ball squat
(*p60*)

☐ Stationary lunge
(*p68*)

☐ Calf raise
(*p71*)

☐ Seated knee
extension (*p72*)

☐ Bent-leg lift
(*p74*)

LEVEL 2 (INTERMEDIATE)

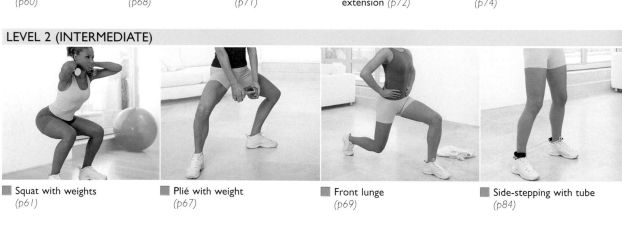

☐ Squat with weights
(*p61*)

☐ Plié with weight
(*p67*)

☐ Front lunge
(*p69*)

☐ Side-stepping with tube
(*p84*)

LEVEL 3 (ADVANCED)

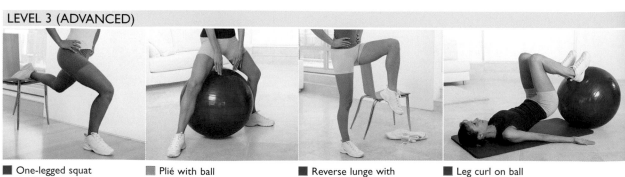

☐ One-legged squat
(*p62*)

☐ Plié with ball
(*p66*)

☐ Reverse lunge with
knee lift (*p70*)

☐ Leg curl on ball
(*p77*)

TRAINING GUIDELINES

- Remember to warm up (pp32–37) before you start and to stretch out (pp86–89) after working the muscles.
- Use proper body alignment and good form.
- Start gently and avoid pain.
- Gradually increase the intensity.

- Use the colour code to guide you in your choice of exercise:
  Beginner: suitable for most people
  Intermediate: requires more strength and coordination
  Advanced: challenges strength and balance

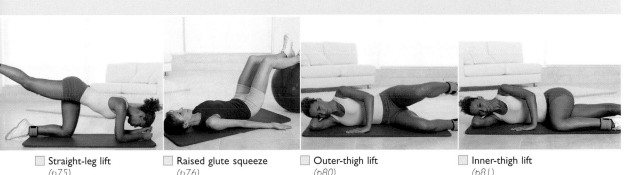

☐ Straight-leg lift (p75)

☐ Raised glute squeeze (p76)

☐ Outer-thigh lift (p80)

☐ Inner-thigh lift (p81)

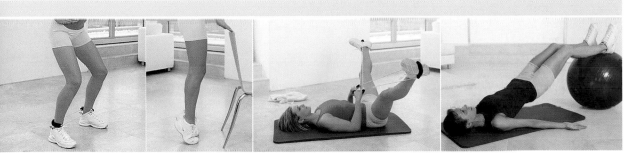

■ Side-step with squat (p84)

■ Calf raise (p71)

■ Scissors with tubes (p85)

■ Ball bridge (p77)

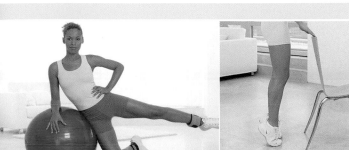

■ Outer-thigh lift on ball (p81)

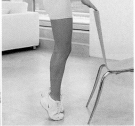

■ Calf raise (p71)

GLUTES & THIGHS: SQUATS 1

The Ball Squat builds up your leg strength and tests your knees before you attempt the Squat with Weights. Leaning some of your body weight against the ball reduces the load on your knees as you come up from the lowest point. You will feel these exercises in your quads first, but if you concentrate on your glutes and hamstrings, you will also feel them at work, lifting and shaping your buttocks.

WEIGHTS & REPETITIONS

Shaping and toning 1–2kg (3–5lb) free weights. Do 15 reps per set.

Bone building 4–6kg (8–12lb) free weights. Do 8–12 reps per set.

☐ BALL SQUAT

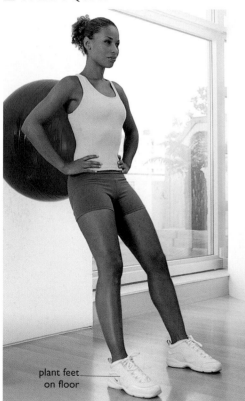

plant feet on floor

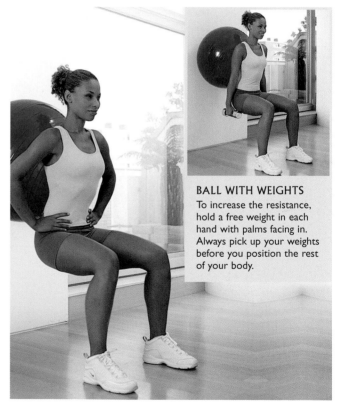

BALL WITH WEIGHTS
To increase the resistance, hold a free weight in each hand with palms facing in. Always pick up your weights before you position the rest of your body.

1 Position the stability ball against the wall so it fits snugly into the natural curve of your spine. Place your hands on your hips. Leaning your weight against the ball, walk your feet forwards until your legs are almost straight.

2 Keeping your back straight, inhale, and slowly bend your knees until your thighs are parallel to the floor, or as far as you can go. Make sure that your knees are directly over your ankles. Pause briefly, then exhale and tighten your buttocks to push back up to the start position.

■ SQUAT WITH WEIGHTS

2 Inhale as you slowly bend your knees to 90 degrees, reaching back with your hips as if you were going to sit down. Allow your torso to lean forwards, but keep your spine straight and your eyes forwards. Pause briefly, then exhale, and tighten your buttocks as you push through your heels to return to the start position.

1 Rest a free weight on each shoulder. Stand with your feet parallel, hip-width apart. Plant your heels on the floor and shift your weight back onto them so that you can lift your toes easily.

keep knees behind toes

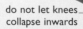

do not let knees collapse inwards

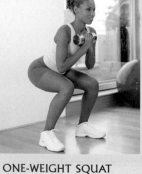

ONE-WEIGHT SQUAT
If you find it easier, hold one heavier weight (2–5kg/5–10lb) at chest height as you perform the exercise. Hug the weight tightly against your body.

GLUTES & THIGHS: SQUATS 2

Working one side of the body at a time – also known as unilateral work – highlights asymmetries between the sides. Right away you can observe which side is stronger, more dominant, stable, and coordinated, and which side needs work. The goal is to develop balance throughout the body. Be sure to work the weaker side first, both to give it mental priority and to be able to match the number of reps you can do on the stronger side.

> **WEIGHTS & REPETITIONS**
> **Shaping and toning** Do 12–15 reps per set.
> **Bone building** 2–4kg (5–8lb) free weights. Do 8–12 reps per set.

■ ONE-LEGGED SQUAT

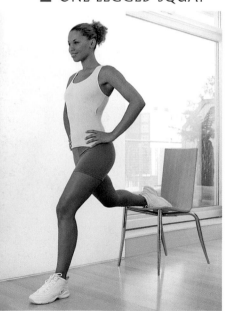

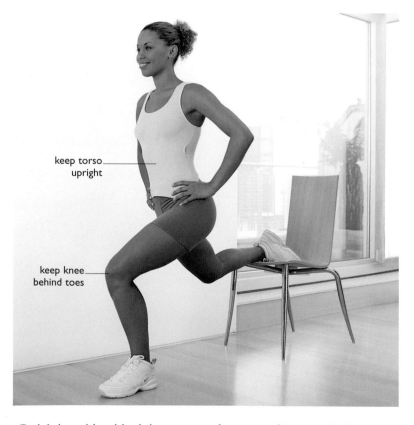

keep torso upright

keep knee behind toes

1 With hands on hips, or holding a free weight in each hand by your sides, palms in, stand a giant step away from a sturdy chair. Place the top of one foot on the chair behind you, then position the front foot with the knee over the ankle. Contract your abdominals to stabilize your torso.

2 Inhale and bend both knees as you lower your hips towards the floor. Keep the front knee behind your toes and your torso upright. Pause briefly, then exhale, and straighten both legs back to the start position. Do all your reps, then switch legs and repeat.

IN THE GYM: THE LEG PRESS 1

The One-Legged Press works the same muscles as the One-Legged Squat – the gluteals, quads, and hamstrings – but in a weight-supported position. The free-standing calisthenic on the opposite page is a weight-bearing exercise that also requires balance and stabilization. The advantage of the leg-press machine is that you can press more weight. Do both if you can.

■ ONE-LEGGED PRESS

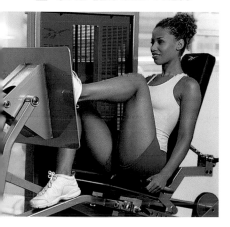

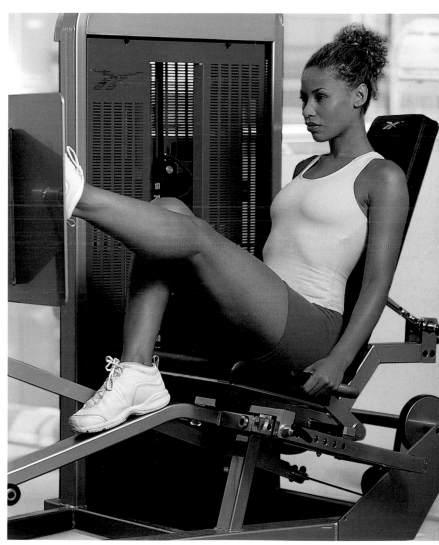

1 Position the seat on the machine so that your left thigh is bent close to your chest. Place your foot on the footplate so that the knee is directly over the ankle. Rest the other leg on the side, safely away from the mechanism of the machine. Grasp the handles with your hands.

WEIGHTS & REPETITIONS

For shaping and toning, set the machine at 18–23kg (40–50lb) and do 12–15 reps per set.

For bone building, set the machine at 27–32kg (60–70lb) and do 8–12 reps per set.

Note: Weights on machines vary widely. Be sure to consult with staff at your gym as to how a particular machine works.

2 Exhale as you extend your leg until it is straight but not stiff. Inhale and slowly bend your knee to 90 degrees, keeping tension in the muscles. Pause, then repeat without resting. Do all your reps, then switch legs and repeat.

IN THE GYM: THE LEG PRESS 2

The Leg Press on the machine offers an alternative to a standing squat. Both exercises work the large muscles of the hips and thighs; however, in the seated position with your weight supported, you can protect your lower back by stabilizing your torso against the seat back and reduce strain on your knees by maintaining precise alignment.

LEG PRESS

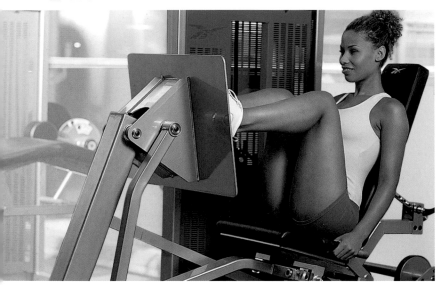

1 Position the seat on the machine so that your thighs are bent close to your chest. Place your feet on the footplate, hip-width apart, with your knees directly over your ankles. Keep your back pressed firmly against the seat back. With your arms by your sides, hold the handles loosely.

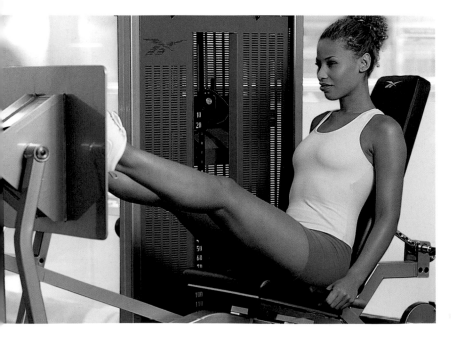

2 Exhale as you extend your legs until they are straight, but not stiff. Inhale as you slowly bend your knees to 90 degrees, keeping tension in the muscles. Pause, then repeat.

WEIGHTS & REPETITIONS FOR MACHINE SHOWN

Leg Press For shaping and toning, set the machine at 36–41kg (80–90lb) and do 12–15 reps. **For bone building**, set the machine at 45–50kg (100–110lb) and do 8–12 reps. **Calf Raise** For shaping and toning, set the machine at 18–23kg (40–50lb). Do 12–15 reps. **For bone building**, set the machine at 27–32kg (60–70lb) and do 8–12 reps. *Note: Weights on machines vary widely. Be sure to consult with staff at your gym as to how a particular machine works.*

■ CALF RAISE

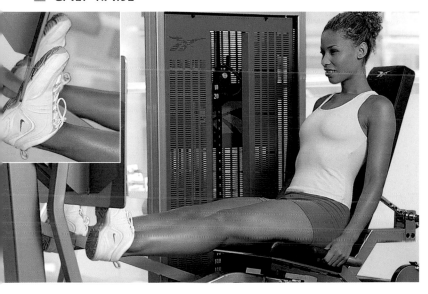

Take advantage of a perfect opportunity to work your lower leg while you are sitting on this machine. The Calf Raise (*see also p71*) helps balance the development of the muscles of the upper leg.

1 With your legs extended, position your feet hip-width apart, the balls of your feet placed on the lower edge of the footplate, with your heels off the plate. With your arms by your sides, hold the handles loosely.

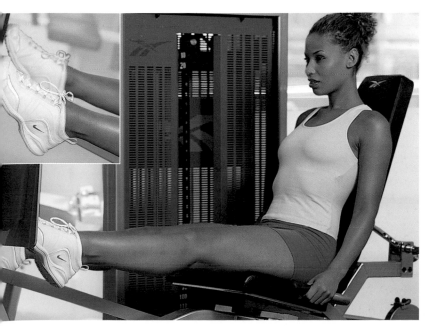

2 Exhale as you slowly push the footplate away with your forefeet. Pause, then inhale as you release the footplate by flexing your feet. Do this in one fluid movement.

GLUTES & THIGHS: PLIÉS

The plié is a variation of the squat. The turned-out position targets the inner thigh, as well as the buttocks, quads, and hamstrings. The key to doing the exercise is to keep the heels down and push through them. If you focus on squeezing the inner thigh and buttocks, you will feel them work as you lift up from the lowest position.

<table>
<tr><td>

WEIGHTS & REPETITIONS

For Plié with Weight 1 ×
2–7kg (5–15lb) free weight. Do
8–15 reps per set.

</td></tr>
</table>

■ PLIÉ WITH BALL

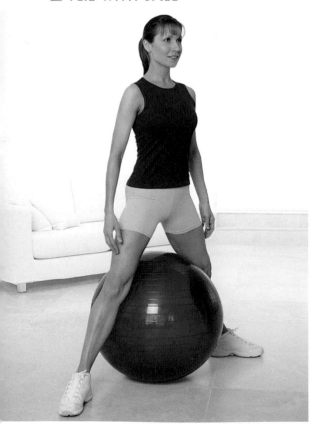

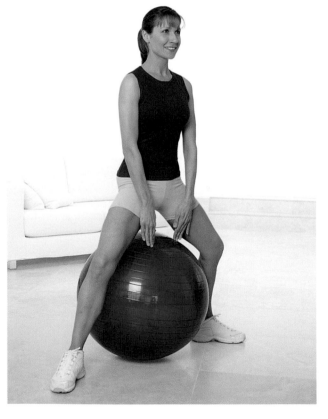

1 Straddle the stability ball. Shift your weight to your heels and turn your legs and feet out from the hips as a unit until your feet are at 45-degree angles. Position the ball so that you can squeeze it hard with the insides of your knees.

2 Keeping your torso upright, inhale as you slowly bend your knees, holding the ball in place with your fingertips. Exhale as you straighten your legs and squeeze the ball with your knees, tightening the inner thighs. Hold for 2–3 seconds, then release. Do 15 reps per set.

■ PLIÉ WITH WEIGHT

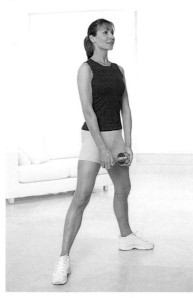

TRAINER'S TIPS
- **A common mistake** is to lean the upper body forwards. Keep your torso upright, and your abdominals contracted.
- **Keep your knees soft** at the top of the movement.
- **As you bend your legs**, don't let your knees roll inwards.
- **Don't let your thighs** go farther than parallel to the floor.

1 Take a wide stance. Shift your weight to your heels and turn your legs and feet out from the hips as a unit until your feet are at 45-degree angles. Hold the free weight straight down in front of you with both hands.

bend knees over toes

push through heels

2 Inhale as you slowly bend your knees until your thighs are parallel to the floor, or as far as they can go. Pause briefly, then exhale as you straighten your legs. Push through your heels and squeeze the inner thighs and buttocks as you lift up.

GLUTES & THIGHS: LUNGES 1

The lunge is a multijoint exercise that strengthens the glutes, quads, and hamstrings. You are bound to feel the quads burning (working) in the front of the thigh first, but the lunge is also working the glutes and hamstrings in one of the best shaping exercises for your buttocks and back of the thigh. Begin with the Stationary Lunge with the feet in a fixed position, and your hand on a chair back for support. Progress to the Front Lunge, which requires balance and stabilization.

WEIGHTS & REPETITIONS

Shaping and toning 1–2kg (3–5lb) free weights. Do 15 reps on each leg per set.

Bone building 4–6kg (8–12lb) free weights. Do 8–12 reps on each leg per set.

◻ STATIONARY LUNGE

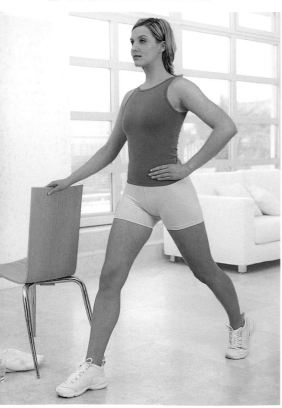 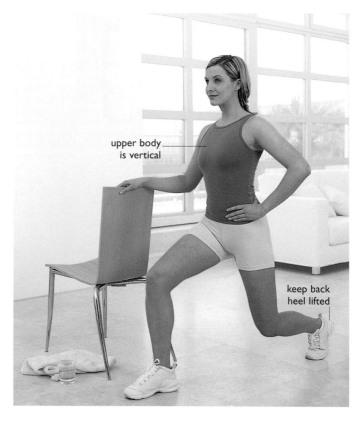

upper body is vertical

keep back heel lifted

1 Stand with your feet parallel, a giant step apart, with your back heel lifted. Keep your hips square to the front and your weight centred evenly between your feet.

2 Inhale as you bend both knees until your back knee is close to the floor and your front knee is directly over the ankle. Exhale as you straighten your legs. The motion is up and down, not forward and backward. Do all your reps, then switch legs and repeat.

■ FRONT LUNGE

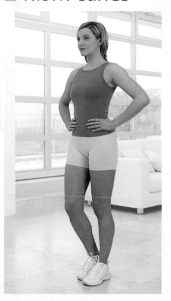

1 Stand in the ready position, feet together, with your weight on your left, supporting leg. Rest your hands lightly on your waist.

ADDING WEIGHTS

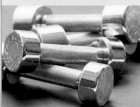

Master the correct form before adding weights. In the Stationary Lunge hold a weight in the hand opposite the front leg. In the Front Lunge, hold a weight in each hand by your sides.

keep knee over ankle

2 Inhale as you step forwards with your right leg and come up on the toes of your back foot. Bend both knees so that the right, front knee is bent directly over the ankle and the back knee is close to the floor. Pause, then exhale to spring back to the start position. Do all your reps, then switch legs and repeat, or alternate sides.

GLUTES & THIGHS: LUNGES 2

Adding variations to basic exercises keeps your workout challenging. The Reverse Lunge with Knee Lift is an advanced lunge that requires you to stabilize on one leg while performing a difficult lunge with the other. It works the same muscles as the lunges on pp68–69, plus the hip flexor. To balance the development of the hips and thighs, it is important to strengthen the lower leg as well. The Calf Raise is a classic exercise for toning the calves.

WEIGHTS & REPETITIONS

For Calf Raise

Shaping and toning 1 × 1–2kg (3–5lb) free weight. Do 12–15 reps on each leg/both legs per set.

Bone building 1 × 4–5kg (8–10 lb) free weight. Do 8–12 reps on each leg/both legs per set.

■ REVERSE LUNGE WITH KNEE LIFT

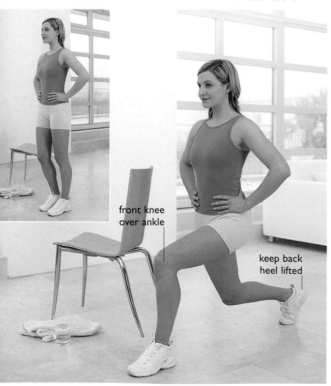

front knee over ankle

keep back heel lifted

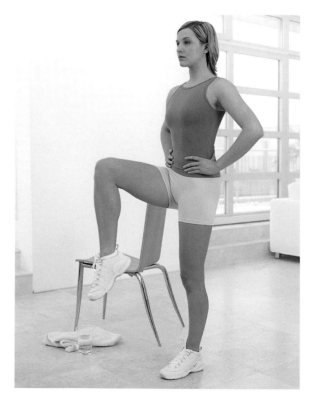

1 Stand near a chair in case you need support, but try not to hold on. Start with both feet together, your hands on your hips. Inhale as you take a giant step back with your right leg and kneel down, bending both knees so that your right knee is close to the floor.

2 Exhale as you straighten your left leg and bring your right knee up to the front, lifting it to hip height. Step back into a reverse lunge, as in Step 1, without stopping at centre. Keep your left, supporting knee soft. Do 12–15 reps, then switch legs and repeat.

■ CALF RAISE

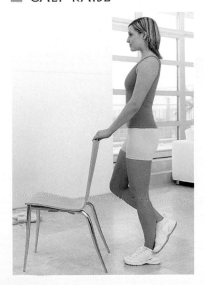

2 Exhale as you lift up on the ball of the working foot as high as you can go. Inhale as you slowly lower the heel back to the floor without resting. Do all your reps, then switch legs and repeat.

1 Stand on one leg, with the opposite toe wrapped around the back of the ankle, consolidating your body weight on the working leg. Rest your hands on the back of a chair for support.

FEEL IT HERE

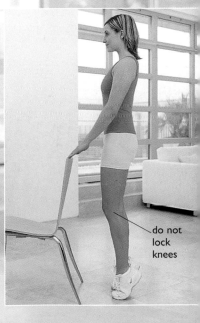

do not lock knees

3 After working one side at a time, work both sides together; exhale as you lift up on the balls of both feet. Pause, then inhale as you lower the heels back to the floor. Repeat 12–15 times. Progress to holding a free weight in one hand.

KNEE EXTENSIONS

Many women develop problems with their knees due to weak quads. Both of these exercises strengthen the quad muscles that run along the front of the thigh, keeping the kneecap tracking properly and reinforcing the knee joint. They are great exercises for beginners who need to build strength before they can progress to higher intensity squats and lunges. They are also classic rehabilitation exercises, since the quads lose strength quickly after a knee injury.

> ## WEIGHTS & REPETITIONS
> **Shaping and toning** 0.5–1kg (1–3lb) ankle weights. Do 15–20 reps on each leg per set.
> **Bone building** 2–4.5kg (5–10lb) ankle weights. Do 8–12 reps on each leg per set.

☐ SEATED KNEE EXTENSION

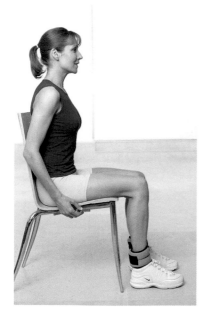

1 Put your ankle weights on first. Sit up tall in a chair, with your legs hip-width apart, your knees bent at a right angle and your feet flat on the floor. Rest your hands on the sides of the chair.

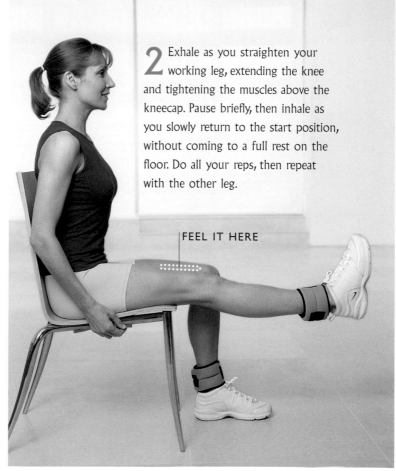

2 Exhale as you straighten your working leg, extending the knee and tightening the muscles above the kneecap. Pause briefly, then inhale as you slowly return to the start position, without coming to a full rest on the floor. Do all your reps, then repeat with the other leg.

FEEL IT HERE

◻ MODIFIED KNEE EXTENSION

This exercise uses a limited range of motion. Add ankle weights when you are ready to increase the resistance.

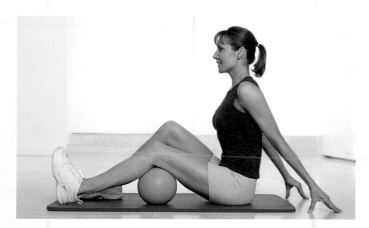

1 Sit up tall on the mat, with your spine straight, your knees bent, and your feet flat on the mat. Put a soft ball (about 19cm/7½in) or a rolled-up towel under your working knee to bring it to a 45-degree angle. Rest your heel on the floor. Place your fingertips on the floor behind you.

2 Exhale as you straighten the working leg, pulling up on the kneecap. Pause briefly, then inhale as you lower the leg slowly to the start position without coming to a full rest on the floor. Do all your reps, then repeat with the other leg.

FEEL IT HERE

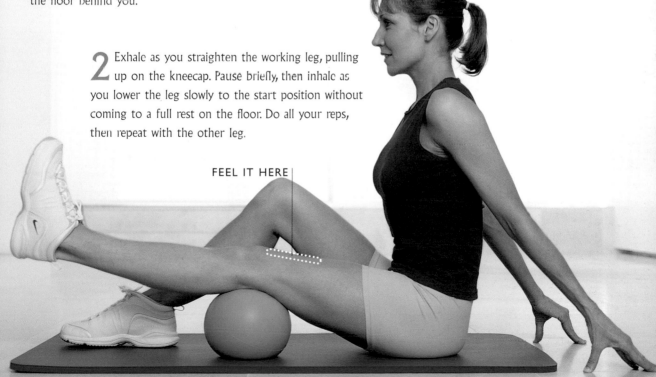

GLUTES & THIGHS: LEG LIFTS

The Bent-Leg Lift targets the glutes, and the straight-leg version works the hamstrings to give a nice shape to the back of the thigh. For shaping and toning with light weights, you will get better results by doing additional sets and reps. If you are just beginning, switch legs after each set; if you are more advanced, do 2–3 sets in a row for each leg. To intensify the work, do a set of 10 reps, then raise the leg one more time and pulse the leg 10 times for a total of 20 reps.

WEIGHTS & REPETITIONS
Shaping and toning 0.5–1kg (1–3lb) ankle weights. Do 15–20 reps on each leg per set.

Bone building 2–4.5kg (5–10lb) ankle weights. Do 8–12 reps on each leg per set.

▢ BENT-LEG LIFT

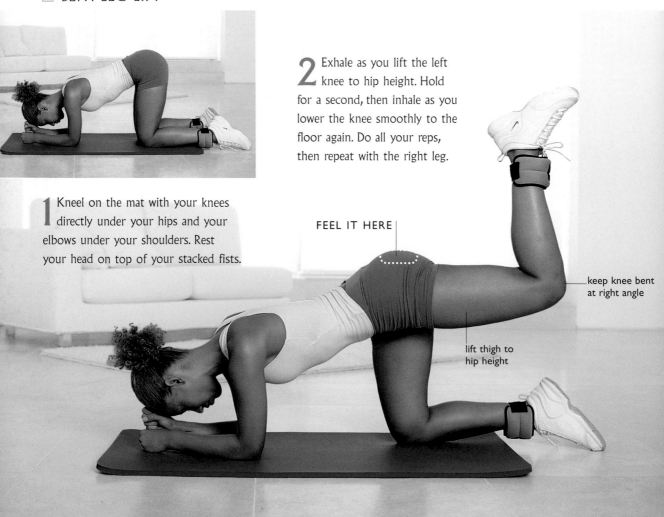

2 Exhale as you lift the left knee to hip height. Hold for a second, then inhale as you lower the knee smoothly to the floor again. Do all your reps, then repeat with the right leg.

1 Kneel on the mat with your knees directly under your hips and your elbows under your shoulders. Rest your head on top of your stacked fists.

FEEL IT HERE

keep knee bent at right angle

lift thigh to hip height

☐ STRAIGHT-LEG LIFT

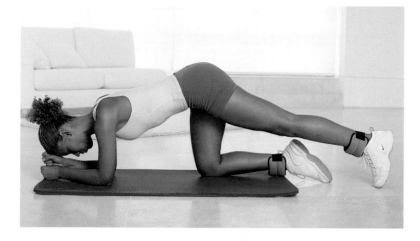

TRAINER'S TIPS

• **Contract your abdominals** to support your lower back and prevent it from arching.

• **Placing your head** on stacked fists ensures proper alignment.

• **Make sure** your working foot is relaxed, not pointed or flexed.

• **Once you begin** a set, do not rest your working leg on the floor. Tap the floor lightly and then lift again immediately.

1 Kneel on the mat as in Bent-Leg Lift, but extend the left leg behind you, toes resting on the floor.

2 Exhale, tighten the hamstrings, and lift your left leg until your thigh is parallel to the floor. Hold for a second, then inhale as you lower the leg smoothly to the floor. Do all your reps, then repeat with the right leg.

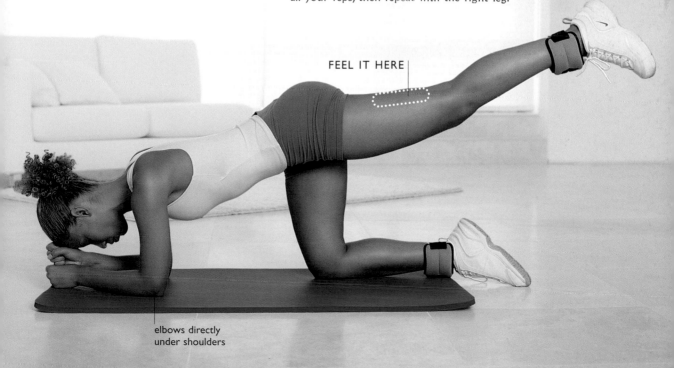

FEEL IT HERE

elbows directly under shoulders

GLUTES & THIGHS: ON THE BALL

These exercises shape the glutes and hamstrings, lifting and strengthening the buttock muscles that support the lower back and toning the back of the thigh. Doing these exercises on the ball also engages the abdominals and spinal extensors as core stabilizers. You will feel the work in the buttocks and back of the thigh.

REPETITIONS

For Ball Bridge Start with 5 reps and progress to 10 reps per set.

☐ RAISED GLUTE SQUEEZE

Both this exercise and the Ball Bridge opposite can be done with your knees bent, feet flat on the floor, or with your heels on the seat of a sturdy chair. Turning the palms up decreases the support of the arms and forces the glutes to work harder.

1 Lie on your back on the mat, knees bent at 90 degrees, with your heels and ankles resting on the stability ball. Place your arms by your sides with the palms up.

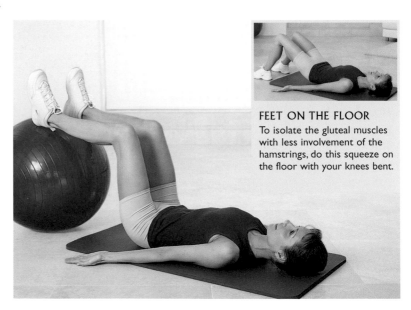

FEET ON THE FLOOR
To isolate the gluteal muscles with less involvement of the hamstrings, do this squeeze on the floor with your knees bent.

2 Press your heels into the ball and squeeze your buttocks tight, lifting them 5–7.5cm (2–3in) off the floor; keep the back of the waist in contact with the floor. Lower your buttocks back to the floor without resting and repeat 15–20 times, then stay in the lifted position and pulse 15–20 times.

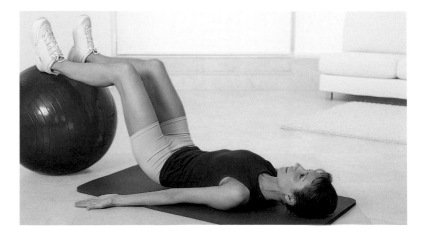

▦ BALL BRIDGE

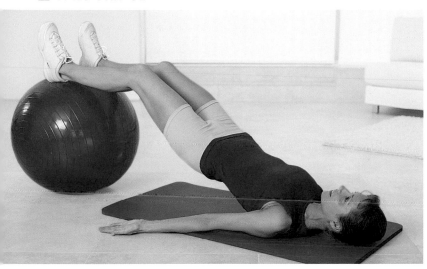

Rest your heels on the ball (or a chair), arms by your sides, palms up. Alternatively, place your feet on the floor, knees bent. Peel your back off the floor, lifting your hips until they form a straight line from the shoulders to the knees. Roll down sequentially through your spine, trying to touch down one vertebra at a time. The biggest challenge is to articulate through the curve in the lower back. Exhale as you lift up on a count of 4, and inhale as you lower down on a count of 4.

▦ LEG CURL ON BALL

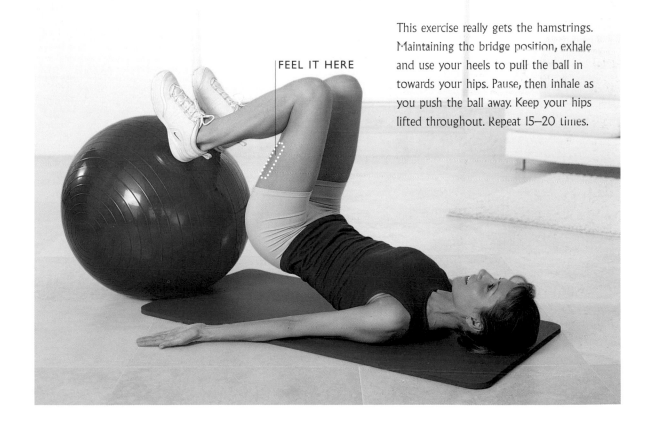

FEEL IT HERE

This exercise really gets the hamstrings. Maintaining the bridge position, exhale and use your heels to pull the ball in towards your hips. Pause, then inhale as you push the ball away. Keep your hips lifted throughout. Repeat 15–20 times.

IN THE GYM: THE PRONE LEG CURL

You can do two great exercises on the prone leg-curl machine to shape the back of the leg. The Hamstring Curl streamlines the rear of the thigh and the buttocks, as does the Back Extension, which also offers the additional benefit of strengthening the spinal extensors. For at-home variations of these exercises, see pp74–77 and the back extensions on pp46–49.

☐ HAMSTRING CURL

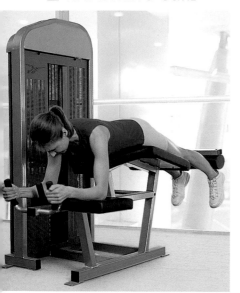

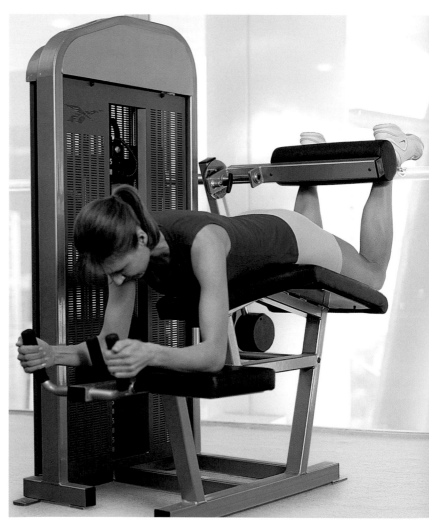

1 Lie face down on the machine, lining your hips up with the bend in the pad. (If your machine is flat, use a rolled towel under your hips to support your lower back.) Position the ankle bar on the back of your ankles and grasp the handles with your hands, resting your elbows on the pads, if they are provided on your machine. Your feet should be relaxed.

2 Tighten your abs and buttocks to prevent your lower back from arching. Keeping your hipbones pressed down evenly against the pad, exhale and bend your knees to 90 degrees, making sure there is no direct pressure on the kneecaps. Pause, then inhale and slowly release to the start position.

WEIGHTS & REPETITIONS FOR MACHINE SHOWN

Hamstring Curl For shaping and toning, set the machine at 9–11kg (20–25lb) and do12–15 reps.
For bone building, set the machine at 14–16kg (30–35lb) and do 8–12 reps.

Back Extension Do 15–20 reps (this is an endurance exercise for everyone).
Note: Weights on machines vary widely. Be sure to consult with staff at your gym as to how a particular machine works.

■ BACK EXTENSION

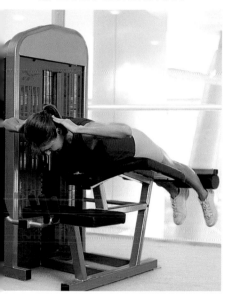

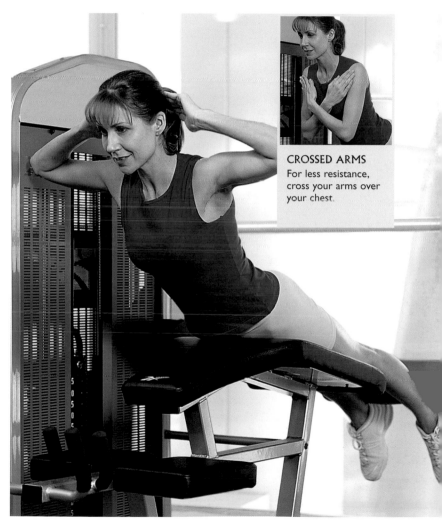

CROSSED ARMS
For less resistance, cross your arms over your chest.

1 Switch the pin to the bottom of the weight stack, making it immovable. Position your ankles under the ankle bar and place your fingertips lightly behind your head. Tighten your buttocks and, using the leverage of your ankles against the bar, lift your torso so that it is off the bench, in line with your hips.

2 Exhale as you continue to tighten your buttocks, raising your torso off the bench. Keep your head and neck in line with your spine, your shoulder blades pulled down and together. Inhale as you slowly return to the start position.

INNER & OUTER THIGHS 1

Most women would rank flabby inner thighs as one of their top three trouble spots (along with a protruding belly and saggy upper arms). The Inner-Thigh Lift will tone and shape the adductor muscles and you will feel them tighten when you do the exercise correctly. The Outer-Thigh Lift gives a nice shape to the hip. Again, for shaping and toning, you will get better results by doing additional sets and reps, and by adding pulses (*see p74*).

WEIGHTS & REPETITIONS

Shaping and toning 0.5–1kg (1–3lb) ankle weights. Do 15–20 reps on each side per set.

Bone building 2–4.5kg (5–10lb) ankle weights. Do 8–12 reps on each side per set.

OUTER-THIGH LIFT

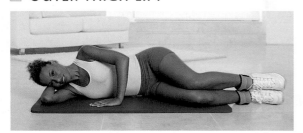

1 Lie on your side on the mat with your hips stacked, your knees bent at a right angle and positioned 45 degrees in front of your body. Rest your head on your bent elbow and use your other hand for support. Roll forwards slightly so that there is a little weight on the supporting arm. (This ensures that you work the outer thigh instead of the front of the thigh).

2 Keeping your knee and ankle level, exhale to lift the top leg to hip height. Pause, then inhale to lower the leg slowly. Repeat without resting. Do all your reps, then turn over and work the other leg. For a variation, straighten the top leg in line with the bottom knee and do another set.

FEEL IT HERE

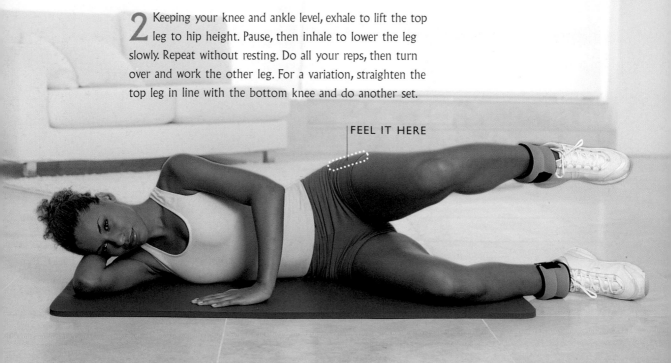

INNER-THIGH LIFT

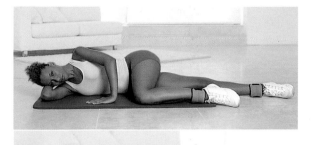

1 Lie on your side on the mat with your hips stacked. Rest your head on your bent elbow and use your other hand for support. Roll forwards slightly so that there is a little weight on the supporting arm. Bend the top knee and rest the leg on the floor, knee in line with your hip.

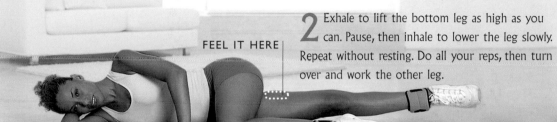

FEEL IT HERE

2 Exhale to lift the bottom leg as high as you can. Pause, then inhale to lower the leg slowly. Repeat without resting. Do all your reps, then turn over and work the other leg.

OUTER-THIGH LIFT ON BALL

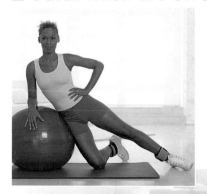

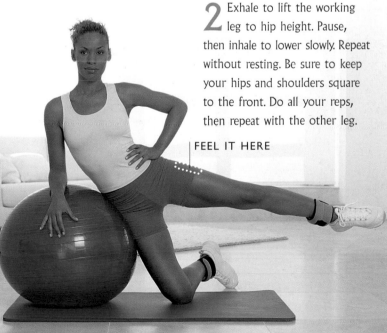

2 Exhale to lift the working leg to hip height. Pause, then inhale to lower slowly. Repeat without resting. Be sure to keep your hips and shoulders square to the front. Do all your reps, then repeat with the other leg.

FEEL IT HERE

1 Kneel, your hips leaning against the ball. Plant your forearm on the ball, your elbow directly under your shoulder. Anchor your shoulder blade and keep your ribs lifted. Place your other hand on your hip. Extend the working leg to the side.

IN THE GYM: HIP ABDUCTOR/ADDUCTOR

These two machines can do the job of hundreds of leg lifts in far fewer moves to tone the inner and the outer thighs. They offer substantial resistance, and are therefore more efficient than floor exercises with ankle weights. In some gyms you will find one machine that you can adjust for both movements.

☐ SEATED HIP ABDUCTION

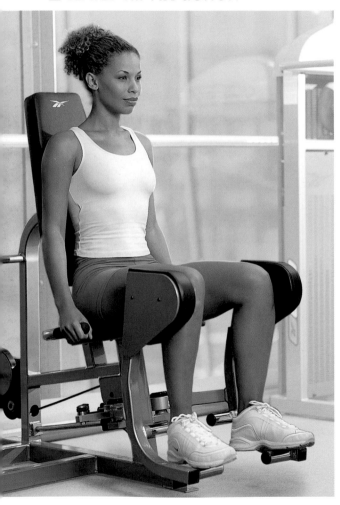 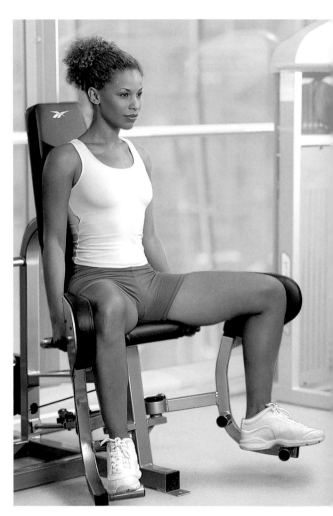

1 Sit with the pads on the outside of your thighs close to your knees. Place your feet on the footplates, legs slightly apart, and make sure that your hips and lower back are firmly against the back support. Grasp the handles with your hands.

2 Exhale as you press your legs open to a comfortable distance. Pause briefly, then inhale as you return slowly to the start position.

WEIGHTS & REPETITIONS FOR MACHINE SHOWN

Hip Abduction For shaping and toning, set the machine at 23–32kg (50–70lb) and do 12–15 reps. **For bone building**, set the machine at 34–43kg (75–95lb) and do 8–12 reps. **Hip Adduction** For shaping and toning, set the machine at 14–18kg (30–40lb) and do 12–15 reps. **For bone building**, set the machine at 20–25kg (45–55lb) and do 8–12 reps. *Note: Weights on machines vary widely. Be sure to consult with staff at your gym as to how a particular machine works.*

☐ SEATED HIP ADDUCTION

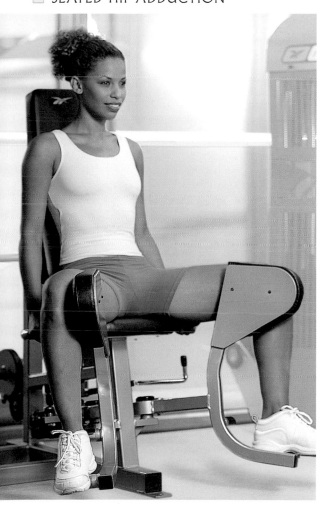

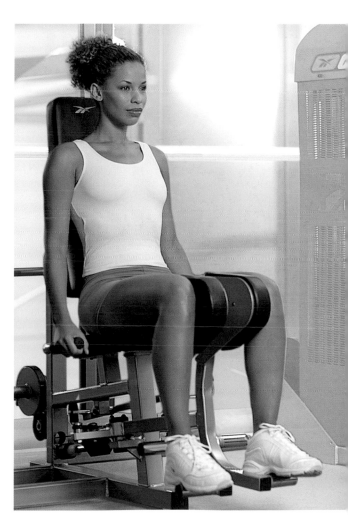

1 Sit with the pads on the inside of your thighs close to your knees. Place your feet on the footplates and press your hips and lower back firmly into the back support. Open the machine so that your legs are slightly more than hip-width apart.

2 Exhale as you pull your legs together until they almost touch. Pause briefly, then inhale as you return slowly to the start position.

INNER & OUTER THIGHS 2

These exercises offer a variation to the ones on pp80-81 for working the inner and the outer thighs. Changing exercises and types of resistance stimulates the muscle with diverse patterns of stress and helps to improve your muscle tone. My clients often ask me to remind them to pack their tubes and bands when they're travelling. You can use stretch bands tied together instead of the tubes.

> ## WEIGHTS & REPETITIONS
>
> **Shaping and toning** Light to medium tubes. Do 15–20 steps/reps per set.
>
> **Bone building** Heavy tubes. Do 8–12 steps/reps per set.

◼ SIDE-STEPPING WITH TUBE

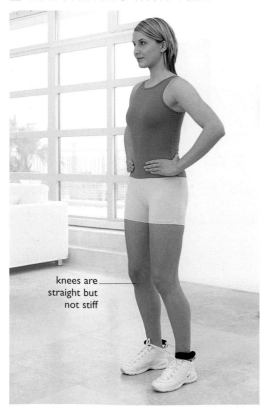

knees are straight but not stiff

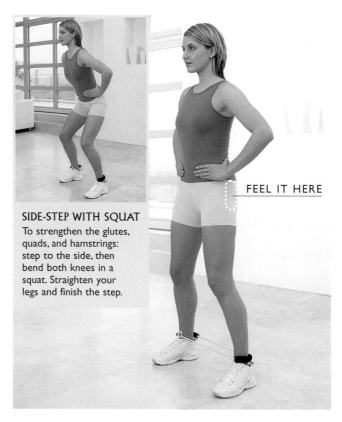

SIDE-STEP WITH SQUAT
To strengthen the glutes, quads, and hamstrings: step to the side, then bend both knees in a squat. Straighten your legs and finish the step.

FEEL IT HERE

1 Stand with the tube around your ankles with the foam cushions on the sides. (Wear thick ankle socks if your ankles need extra protection.) If you have knee problems, place the tube above your knees. Rest your hands on your hips.

2 Separate your legs until you feel tension in the tube. Step to the right, keeping your right, leading leg straight, then follow with your left leg, keeping the tube taut. Continue side-stepping to the right until you have done all your reps, then change direction and lead with your left leg.

■ SCISSORS WITH TUBES

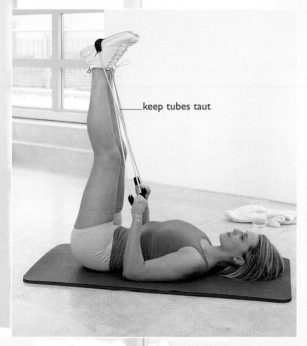

keep tubes taut

TRAINER'S TIPS

• **Keep tension** in the tube throughout in the Side-Step and do not let it go slack.

• **For Scissors**, make sure that each tube is securely anchored in the arch of your shoe.

• **Pull the tubes** taut and hold the handles stationary, in close to your body.

1 You will need two tubes for this exercise. Lie on your back on the mat with your legs straight in the air. Loop a tube around the arch of each foot and hold it with the opposite hand so that the handles are crossed. Hold the foam cushions in close to your body to anchor the tubes.

2 Use your upper-body strength to prevent tension in the neck and shoulders. Without moving your hands, inhale as you open your legs slowly. Exhale as you pull your legs together against the resistance of the tubes.

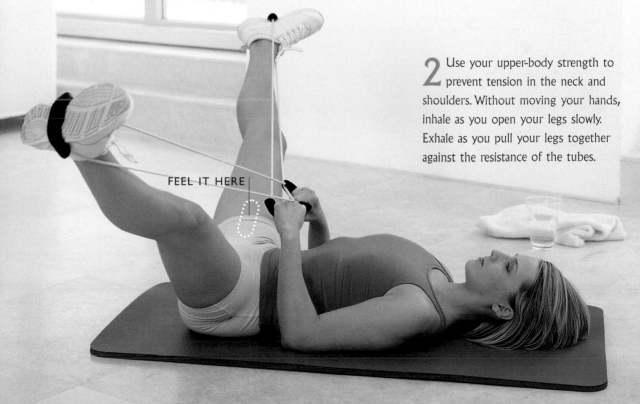

FEEL IT HERE

STANDING LEG STRETCHES

Most of us do not stretch the large muscles in our legs often enough to counteract the daily stresses of prolonged sitting or standing. Go into each of the following stretches until you feel a gentle pull (but not pain) in the muscle. Hold the stretch for 20–30 seconds without bouncing, allowing time for the muscle to lengthen. Breathe into the stretch, using the exhale to move deeper into the position.

☐ CALF STRETCH

☐ HIP-FLEXOR STRETCH

☐ QUAD STRETCH

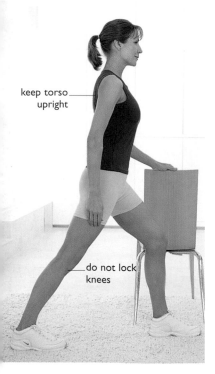

keep torso upright

do not lock knees

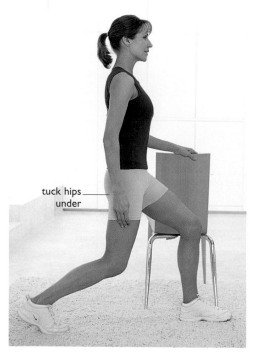

tuck hips under

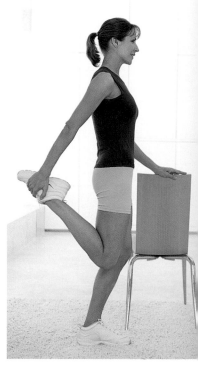

Stand with your feet together and place your left hand on a chair back for support. Take a giant step back with your right leg and press the heel into the floor. Bend your left knee over your ankle. Feel the stretch in the back of the calf.

From the previous position, come up on the toes of your back foot, bend the back knee towards the floor, and press the bottom of the pelvis forwards. Keep the left knee directly over the ankle. Feel the stretch in the front of the right hip.

Stand on your left leg with the knee soft. Bend the right leg and, holding the foot or ankle, bring the heel towards the buttocks. Feel the stretch along the front of the thigh. To intensify the stretch, press the bottom of the pelvis forwards.

HAMSTRING STRETCH

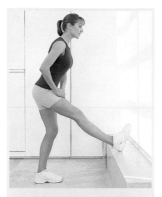

STRETCH ON SUPPORT
Intensify the hamstring stretch by propping your foot up on a low support. The action of the stretch is again to flex forwards from the hip.

keep upper back straight

maintain neutral spine alignment

Stand on your left leg, with the knee bent. Extend your right leg to the front, and rest your heel on the floor, with the toe pointing to the ceiling. Bend forwards from the hip, keeping your upper body in proper alignment. Feel the stretch in your hamstrings. Turn around to perform the sequence of stretches on the left leg.

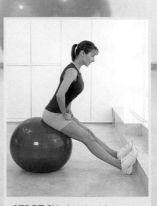

STRETCH ON BALL
This is a great stretch. Sit on the stability ball and prop your feet up against a wall, toes pointing to the ceiling. Sit up tall, then lean forwards with your spine straight, reaching back with your hips.

FLOOR LEG STRETCHES

Stretching the muscles of the upper leg increases mobility of the hip joint and reduces stiffness that may come from lack of use. It also promotes muscle balance around the pelvis, which keeps it in proper alignment and reduces tightness in the lower back. Do this trio of stretches in sequence. It is best to coax the muscle into lengthening by being patient, rather than trying to force a stretch too quickly, which may strain the muscle. Perform these stretches on a mat or a well-padded surface.

■ INNER-THIGH STRETCH

Lie on your back with your feet in the air, soles together, knees out to the sides. Reach through your legs to grasp an ankle with each hand and use your elbows to press open the inner thighs. If you are not flexible enough in the upper body to do this, keep your hands on top of your ankles, and press your elbows into your knees instead.

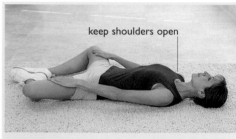

keep shoulders open

DIAMOND STRETCH
If you are not accustomed to stretching the inner thigh, begin by lying on your back with the soles of your feet together on the floor, knees open. Use your hands on your inner thighs to deepen the stretch gently.

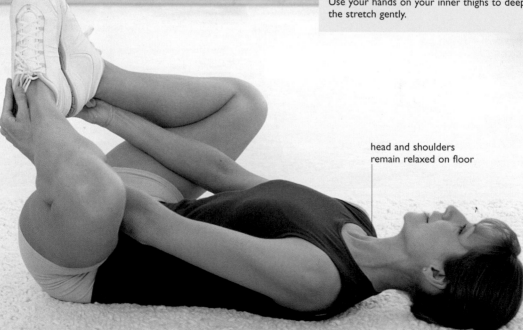

head and shoulders remain relaxed on floor

☐ OUTER-THIGH STRETCH

Lie on your back with your knees bent, feet flat on the floor. Cross your left ankle over the right knee and reach behind the right thigh with both hands, gently pulling your leg towards you. Hold for 30 seconds and repeat on the other side.

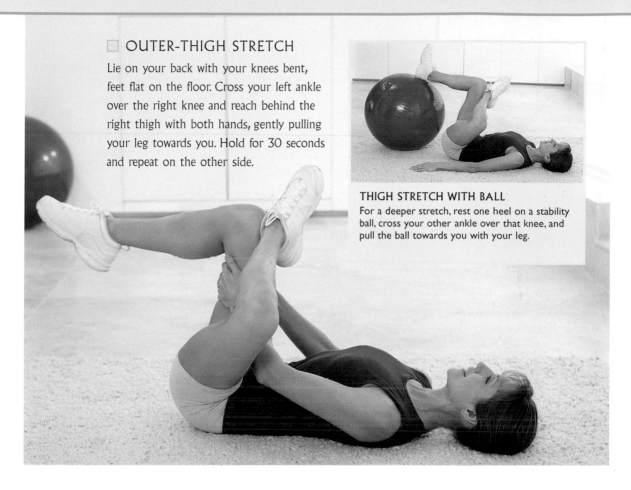

THIGH STRETCH WITH BALL
For a deeper stretch, rest one heel on a stability ball, cross your other ankle over that knee, and pull the ball towards you with your leg.

☐ GLUTE STRETCH

From the Outer-Thigh Stretch, release your hands, slide your knees together just as you were, and hug both knees into your chest. Hold for 30 seconds and repeat on the other side.

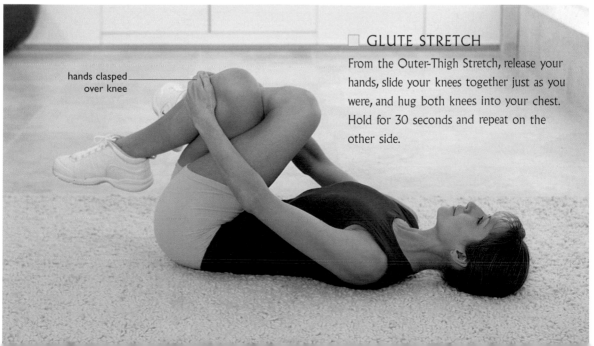

hands clasped over knee

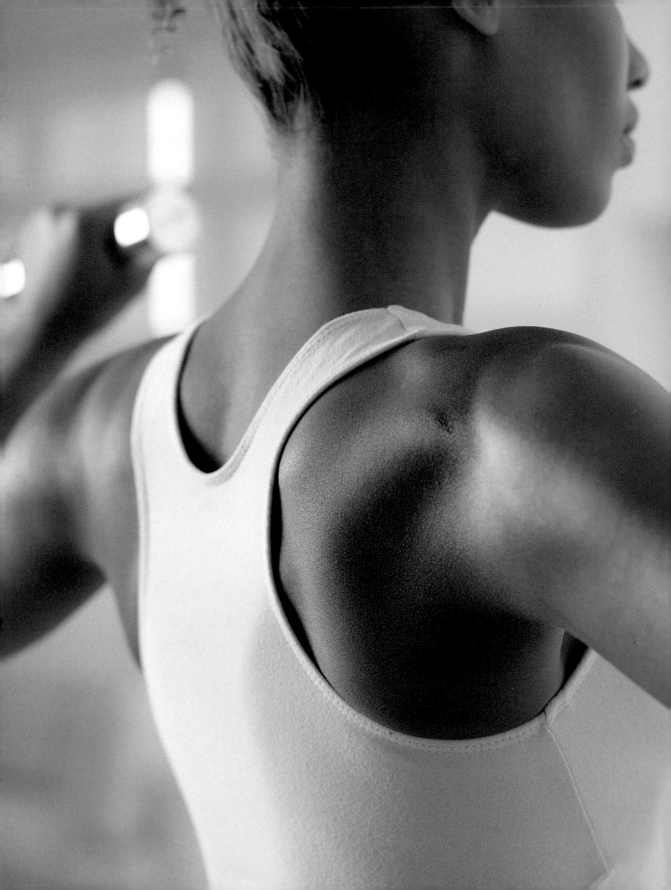

UPPER BODY PROGRAMME

In terms of major muscle groups, the legs are followed in size by the muscles of the back, then the chest, shoulders, and arms, in that order. Most women are weak and undeveloped in their upper bodies. Doing upper-body exercises will improve the muscle tone and appearance of this whole area, as well as enhance your posture and bearing. In addition, they will help to balance out the proportions of your lower body, particularly if you are pear shaped. If you are afraid of appearing too big in the shoulders and arms, for nice definition follow the shaping and toning guidelines.

"I'm constantly reminded of the practical benefits of my training sessions in my everyday life. Whether it's lifting a heavy roasting pan out of the oven or climbing stairs without getting winded, I know that my efforts are paying off." *Erica S.*

PROGRAMMES AT A GLANCE

Work through the programmes below, starting with Level 1 and building up to Level 3. Alternatively, pick an exercise for the back, one for the chest, one for the shoulders, and one for the arms to add to your whole-body programme of 8–10 exercises. The Level 2 programme uses body weight and bands only, which also makes it highly portable.

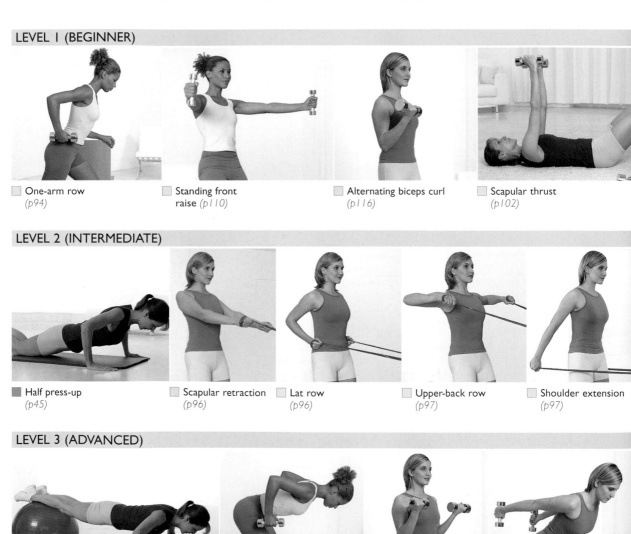

LEVEL 1 (BEGINNER)

☐ One-arm row *(p94)*

☐ Standing front raise *(p110)*

☐ Alternating biceps curl *(p116)*

☐ Scapular thrust *(p102)*

LEVEL 2 (INTERMEDIATE)

■ Half press-up *(p45)*

☐ Scapular retraction *(p96)*

☐ Lat row *(p96)*

☐ Upper-back row *(p97)*

☐ Shoulder extension *(p97)*

LEVEL 3 (ADVANCED)

■ Full press-up on ball *(p45)*

■ Bent-over lat row *(p95)*

■ Biceps "21s" *(p117)*

■ Unsupported triceps kickback *(p119)*

TRAINING GUIDELINES

- Remember to warm up (pp32–37) before you start and to stretch out (pp122–123) after working the muscles.
- Use proper body alignment and good form.
- Start gently and avoid pain.
- Gradually increase the intensity.

- Use the colour code to guide you in your choice of exercise:

  Beginner: suitable for most people

  ▨ Intermediate: requires more strength and coordination

  ▪ Advanced: challenges strength and balance

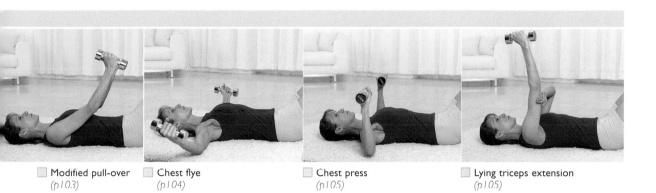

☐ Modified pull-over (p103) ☐ Chest flye (p104) ☐ Chest press (p105) ☐ Lying triceps extension (p105)

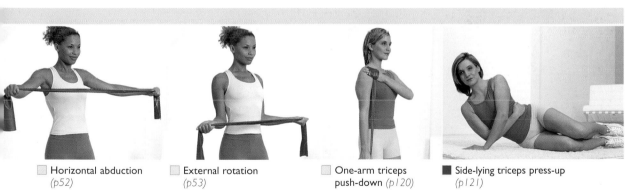

☐ Horizontal abduction (p52) ☐ External rotation (p53) ☐ One-arm triceps push-down (p120) ▪ Side-lying triceps press-up (p121)

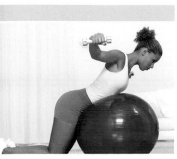

▪ "Ys" and "Ts" on ball (p114)

FOR THE SHOULDERS

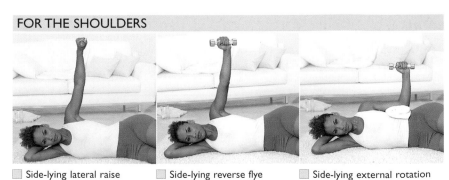

☐ Side-lying lateral raise (p111) ☐ Side-lying reverse flye (p112) ☐ Side-lying external rotation (p112)

THE BACK: LATISSIMUS DORSI

Your lats are the broad muscle of the midback that give it a defined "V" shape, making your waist and hips look slimmer. These exercises firm up the sides of your back and trim the bulges around your bra strap for a sleeker line in bathing suits and sweaters. Training the lats gives more power to your golf swing and swimming stroke. It improves posture, most notably in sports that rely on leg power, such as running, when there is a tendency to hunch the upper body.

> ### WEIGHTS & REPETITIONS
> **Shaping and toning** 2–4kg (5–8lb) free weights. Do 12–15 reps on each side per set.
>
> **Bone building** 5–7kg (10–15lb) free weights. Do 8–12 reps on each side per set.

☐ ONE-ARM LAT ROW

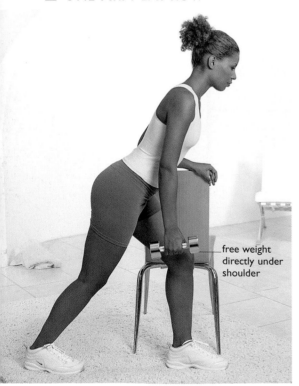

free weight directly under shoulder

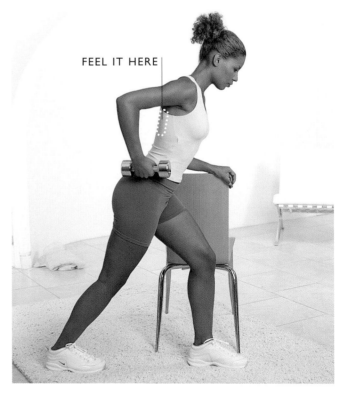

FEEL IT HERE

1 Place your left hand on a chair back for support. Step back with your right foot to stand in a staggered lunge position, your left knee bent over the ankle. Hold a free weight in your right hand, arm straight, palm facing in.

2 Draw your right shoulder blade towards the spine. You can hold this position during the entire exercise or do it at the start of each rep. Exhale as you bend your elbow to 90 degrees, pulling the weight up to your waist. Inhale as you slowly return to the start position. Do all your reps, then switch arms and repeat.

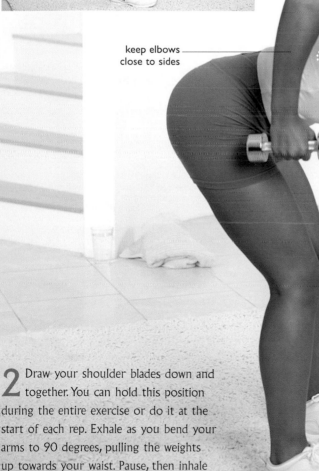

keep knees
slightly bent

■ BENT-OVER LAT ROW

This advanced variation requires enough strength in the torso to stabilize in the bent-over position, with the spine straight and the natural curve in the lower back.

1 Stand with your feet hip-width apart. Hold a free weight in each hand, arms at your sides, palms facing in. Bend forwards from the hips until your back is to the ceiling and your arms hang straight down under your shoulders. Keep your nose down.

keep elbows
close to sides

FEEL IT HERE

2 Draw your shoulder blades down and together. You can hold this position during the entire exercise or do it at the start of each rep. Exhale as you bend your arms to 90 degrees, pulling the weights up towards your waist. Pause, then inhale as you straighten your arms slowly to the start position.

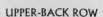

UPPER-BACK ROW

To target the trapezius, rhomboids, and posterior deltoid: draw your shoulder blades down and together, then bend your elbows out to the sides in line with your shoulders, your palms facing back.

FULL TREATMENT FOR THE BACK

The band exercises work the same muscles as the free-weight exercises on pp94–95 and p103, but with a different type of resistance. This is one of my favourite exercise series because it works much of the vital musculature of the back in an easy sequence. Start each exercise by putting a little tension in the band and keeping it taut throughout the movement.

☐ SCAPULAR RETRACTION

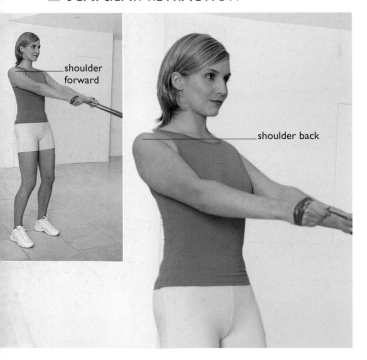

shoulder forward

shoulder back

This works the rhomboid and midtrapezius muscles. It is a very small movement. Tie the middle of the band to a sturdy door knob. Make a knot at each end to form a loop to hold onto with a secure grip or attach ready-made foam handles. Stand with your arms extended, palms facing in, holding one end of the band in each hand. Keep your elbows straight and squeeze the shoulder blades down and together. Hold for a second, then release.

☐ LAT ROW

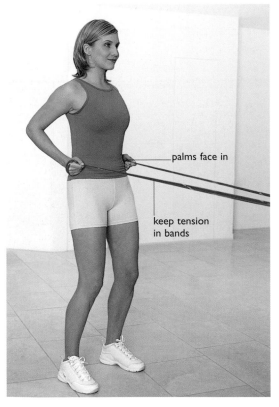

palms face in

keep tension in bands

To work the lats and posterior deltoid: hold the band with your arms extended in front of you, palms facing in. Squeeze the shoulder blades down and together. Exhale as you pull the band into the sides of your waist. Inhale as you release the band.

☐ UPPER-BACK ROW

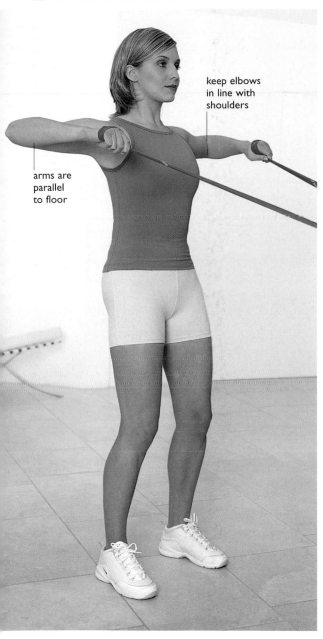

keep elbows
in line with
shoulders

arms are
parallel
to floor

☐ SHOULDER EXTENSION

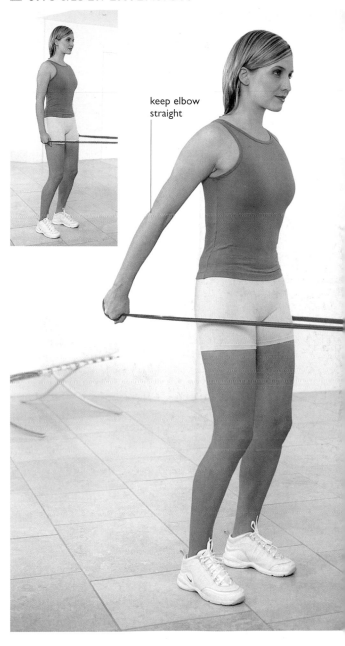

keep elbow
straight

To work the rhomboids, trapezius, and posterior deltoid: hold the band with your arms extended, palms down. Squeeze the shoulder blades down and together. Exhale as you pull the band to shoulder height, bending the elbows out to the sides. Inhale as you release the band.

To work the lats and posterior deltoid: stand with your arms at your sides, holding the band at hip height, palms facing in. Exhale as you pull the band behind you, keeping your elbows straight but not stiff. Pause, then inhale to release the band to the midline of your body.

IN THE GYM: THE LAT PULL-DOWN 1

The lat pull-down machine offers a powerful alternative to working the latissimus dorsi with free weights and bands as shown on pp94–95 and p96. You can lift more weight and target the muscle from a variety of positions. The results – a stronger, straighter back, better posture, and improved sports performance.

☐ SEATED FRONT PULL-DOWN: OVERHAND GRIP

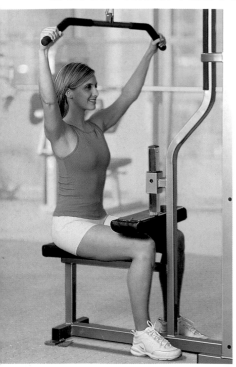

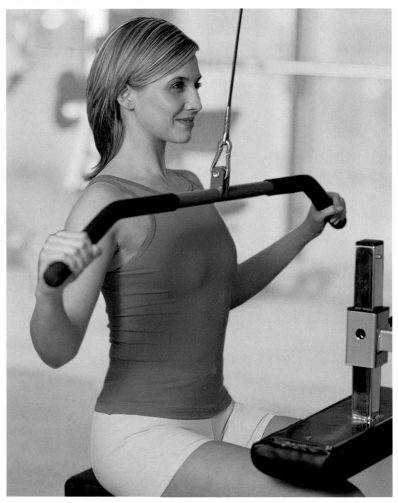

1 Stand with your legs straddling the seat of the lat pull-down. Grasp the bar with both hands in an overhand grip, hands slightly wider than shoulder-width apart. Sit down, holding the bar above your chest with your arms extended, your knees secured under the pad.

2 Draw your shoulder blades down and together. Keeping your back straight and chest lifted, exhale and pull the bar down to the top of your chest, bringing your elbows into your sides so that they point towards the floor. Pause briefly, then inhale, and slowly release to the start position.

WEIGHTS & REPETITIONS FOR MACHINE SHOWN

Overhand Grip For shaping and toning, set the machine at 11–16kg (25–35lb) and do 12–15 reps. **For bone building**, set the machine at 18–23kg (40–50lb) and do 8–12 reps.
Underhand Grip For shaping and toning, set the machine at 14–18kg (30–40lb) and do 12–15 reps. **For bone building**, set at 20–25kg (45–55lb) and do 8–12 reps.

Note: Weights on machines vary widely. Be sure to consult with staff at your gym as to how a particular machine works.

☐ SEATED FRONT PULL-DOWN: UNDERHAND GRIP

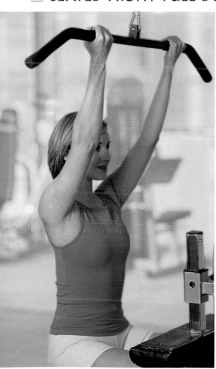

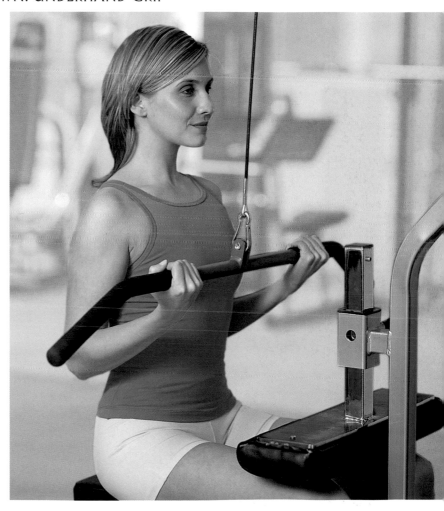

1 Stand with your legs straddling the seat of the lat pull-down. Take the bar with both hands in an underhand grip, hands shoulder-width apart. Sit down with your arms extended overhead, holding the bar above your chest, your knees secured under the pad.

2 Draw your shoulder blades down and together. Keeping your back straight and chest lifted, exhale as you pull the bar down to the middle of your chest, drawing your elbows in close to your sides so that they point behind you. Pause briefly, then inhale as you slowly release the bar to the start position.

IN THE GYM: THE LAT PULL-DOWN 2

The Standing Lat Row mimics the movement in the Seated Front Pull-Down (*p99*) and in the Lat Row with the band (*p96*). The Standing Straight-Arm Pull-Down uses the same action as the Shoulder Extension on p97 and the Modified Pull-over on p103. You will have to lighten the weights on the machine for the standing position. Use an attachment with handles or the bar.

■ STANDING LAT ROW

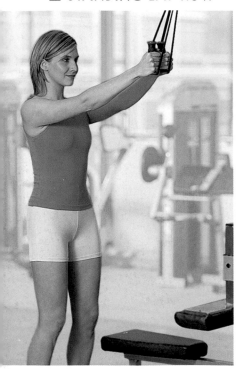

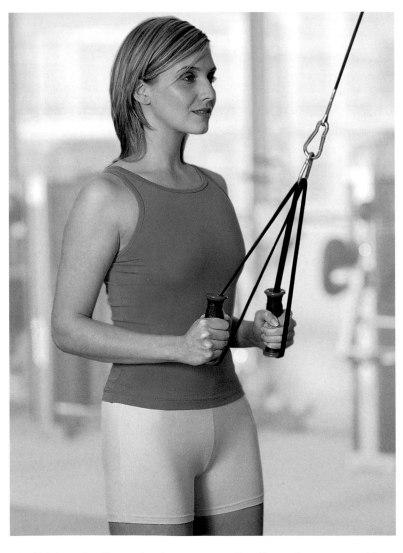

1 Stand with your feet parallel, hip-width apart, knees soft. Grasp the handles of the attachment with your palms facing in, arms extended above shoulder level. Draw your shoulder blades down and together. Contract your abdominals to stabilize the torso.

2 Exhale and pull your hands into your waist, elbows close to your sides and pointing back. Hold for a second, then inhale as you release the handles slowly to the start position.

WEIGHTS & REPETITIONS FOR MACHINE SHOWN

Lat Row For shaping and toning, set the machine at 11–14kg (25–30lb) and do 12–15 reps. **For bone building**, set the machine at 16–18kg (35–40lb), and do 8–12 reps. **Straight-Arm Pull-Down** For shaping and toning, set

the machine at 7–9kg (15–20lb) weights. Do 12–15 reps. **For bone building**, set at 11–14kg (25–30lb) and do 8–12 reps. *Note: Weights on machines vary widely. Be sure to consult with staff at your gym as to how a particular machine works.*

■ STANDING STRAIGHT-ARM PULL-DOWN

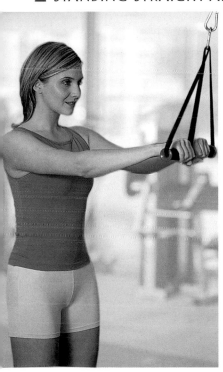

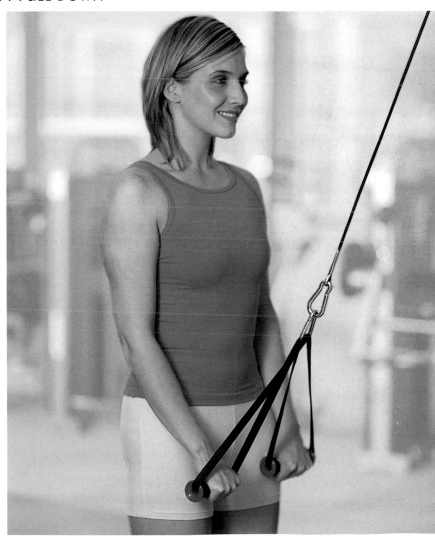

1 Stand with your feet parallel, hip-width apart, your knees soft, at arms' length away from the machine. With palms facing down, pull the handles to the start position at shoulder level. Your arms should be straight but not stiff. Draw your shoulder blades down and together. Contract your abdominals to stabilize your torso.

2 Exhale and, keeping your arms straight, pull the handles down to the front of your thighs in one fluid motion. Hold for a second, then inhale as you release the handles slowly to the start position.

THE CHEST: PECTORALIS MAJOR

Although the main focus of this exercise series is the chest (pectoralis major) to firm the bustline, you are also in the ideal lying position to work the shoulder blades (*Scapular Thrust*) and the triceps (*Lying Triceps Extension, p105*). The Chest Flye (*p104*) works the pecs with the anterior deltoid to firm the area in front of the armpit. The Chest Press (*p105*) brings in the triceps as well to tone the back of the arm.

WEIGHTS & REPETITIONS

Shaping and toning 1–2kg (3–5lb) free weights. Do 12–15 reps per set.

Bone building 4–6kg (8–12lb) free weights. Do 8–12 reps per set.

☐ SCAPULAR THRUST

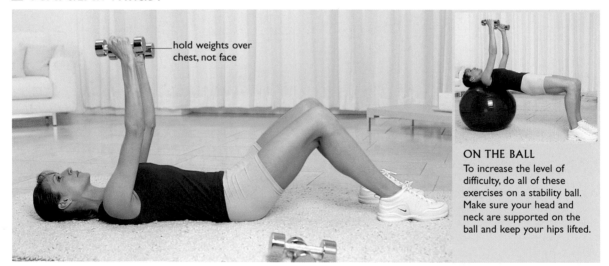

hold weights over chest, not face

ON THE BALL
To increase the level of difficulty, do all of these exercises on a stability ball. Make sure your head and neck are supported on the ball and keep your hips lifted.

1 To work the serratus anterior: lie on your back with your knees bent. Hold a free weight in each hand, palms facing in. Extend your arms to the ceiling so that the weights are over your chest. Anchor your shoulder blades.

2 Exhale as you lift your shoulder blades off the floor, gently thrusting the weights towards the ceiling. Inhale to return. Alternate arms or do both arms together.

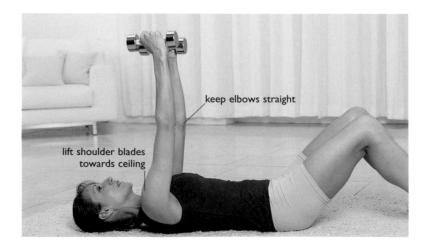

keep elbows straight

lift shoulder blades towards ceiling

☐ MODIFIED PULL-OVER

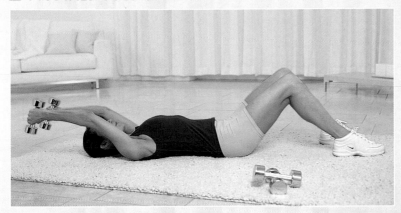

This is my favourite exercise to transition from back to chest work because is it trains both the lats and the pectoralis major.

1 From the start position on the opposite page, anchor your shoulder blades and inhale to lower both free weights overhead towards the floor without touching it. Keep your arms shoulder-width apart.

2 Exhale and pull the weights over your chest to just above your waistline (this is the exertion). Pause, then inhale to lower the weights slowly overhead. If you find this difficult, to start you can do the move holding the weights together or use one weight (2kg/5lb) held with both hands. For a bone-building variation, hold one 6kg (12lb) free weight, or heavier if you can manage.

TRAINER'S TIPS

- **Draw your shoulder blades** down before you move.
- **Keep your arms** straight but not stiff.
- **When you lower** the weights overhead, do not arch your lower back, keep it to the floor.
- **Make the movements** smooth and fluid.

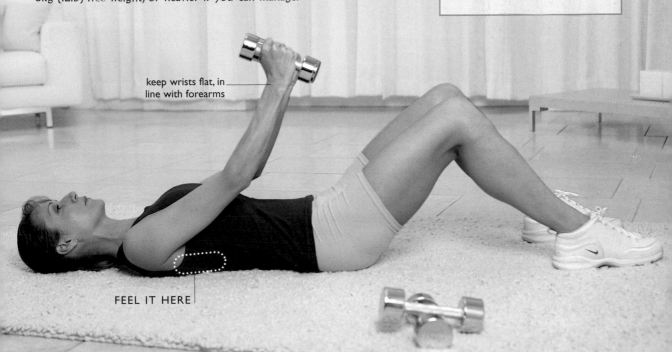

keep wrists flat, in line with forearms

FEEL IT HERE

☐ CHEST FLYE

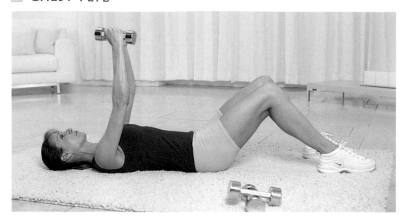

1 To work the pectoralis major and the anterior deltoid: lie on your back with your knees bent, feet flat on the floor. Hold a free weight in each hand, palms facing in, and extend your arms to the ceiling so that the weights are over your chest, not your face. Round your elbows as if you were hugging a tree. Anchor your shoulder blades.

2 Inhale and slowly open your arms out to the sides, moving from the shoulder and keeping your elbows bent at a constant angle. Your upper arms should momentarily touch the floor; your forearms should not. Exhale as you lift your arms back to the start position (this is the exertion).

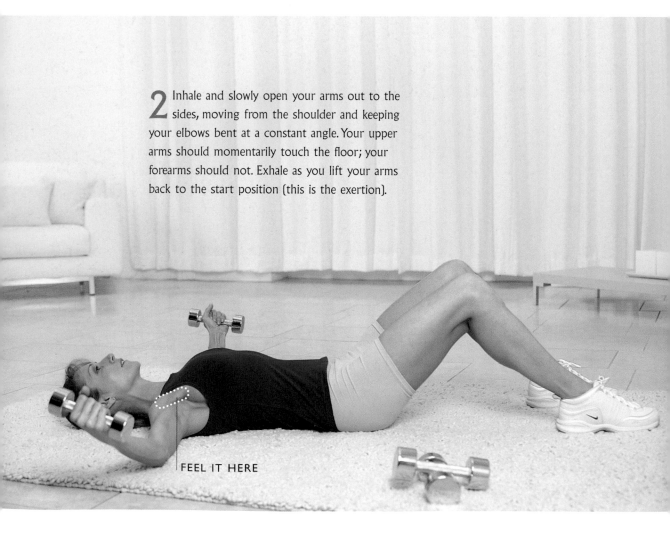

FEEL IT HERE

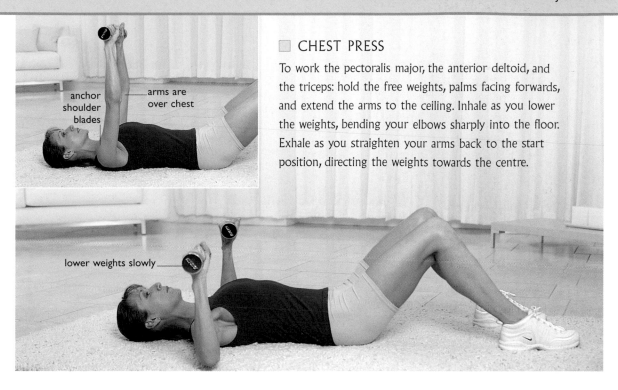

anchor shoulder blades

arms are over chest

lower weights slowly

☐ CHEST PRESS

To work the pectoralis major, the anterior deltoid, and the triceps: hold the free weights, palms facing forwards, and extend the arms to the ceiling. Inhale as you lower the weights, bending your elbows sharply into the floor. Exhale as you straighten your arms back to the start position, directing the weights towards the centre.

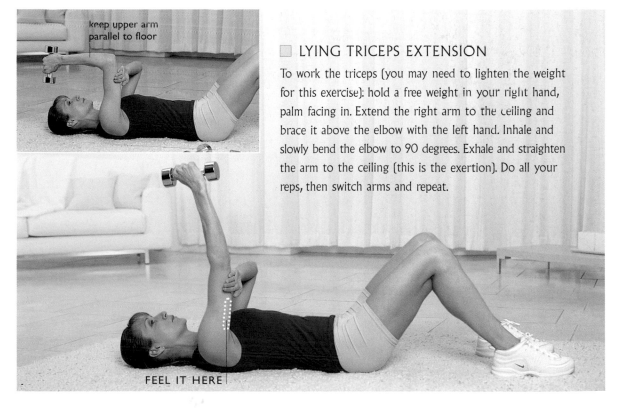

keep upper arm parallel to floor

☐ LYING TRICEPS EXTENSION

To work the triceps (you may need to lighten the weight for this exercise): hold a free weight in your right hand, palm facing in. Extend the right arm to the ceiling and brace it above the elbow with the left hand. Inhale and slowly bend the elbow to 90 degrees. Exhale and straighten the arm to the ceiling (this is the exertion). Do all your reps, then switch arms and repeat.

FEEL IT HERE

IN THE GYM: THE CHEST PRESS

The chest-press machine can be used in addition to free weights (*see Chest Press, p105*) to firm the muscles that support the breasts, tone the front of the shoulder, and sculpt the back of the upper arm. You can also use the machine to strengthen the serratus anterior (*see Scapular Thrust, p102*), the muscle that prevents the shoulder blade from winging out.

☐ SCAPULAR THRUST

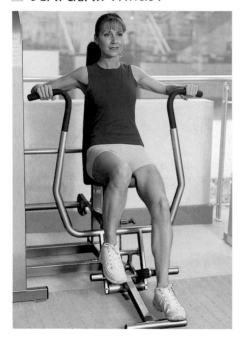

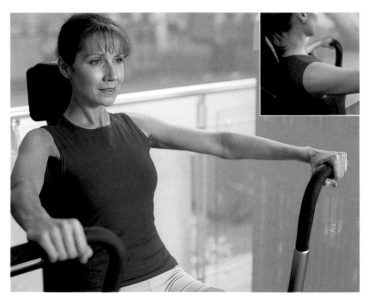

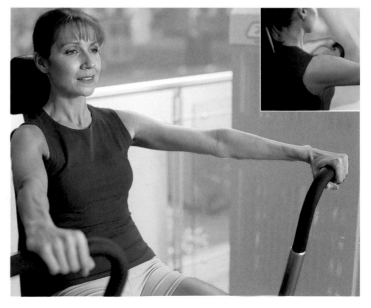

To work the serratus anterior: sit with your back against the padded back support, the seat adjusted so that the knees are bent at a right angle. Use the foot bar to bring the handles forwards (*above*) to ensure that the elbows are not behind the body in a loaded position, putting strain on the shoulder. Extend the arms to the front, elbows straight but not stiff (*top right*). Separate the shoulder blades (*bottom right*), pushing the handles forwards 5–7.5cm (2–3in). Release by bringing the shoulder blades together.

WEIGHTS & REPETITIONS FOR MACHINE SHOWN

Scapular Thrust Set the machine at 9–14kg (20–30lb) and do 15–20 reps (this is an endurance exercise for everyone).

Chest Press For shaping and toning, set the machine at

9–11kg (20–25lb) and do 12–15 reps. **For bone building**, set the machine at 14–16kg (30–35lb) and do 8–12 reps.

Note: Weights on machines vary widely. Be sure to consult with staff at your gym as to how a particular machine works.

☐ CHEST PRESS

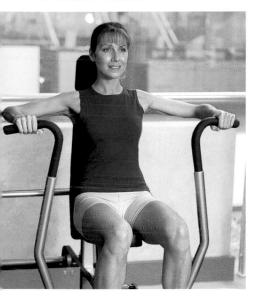

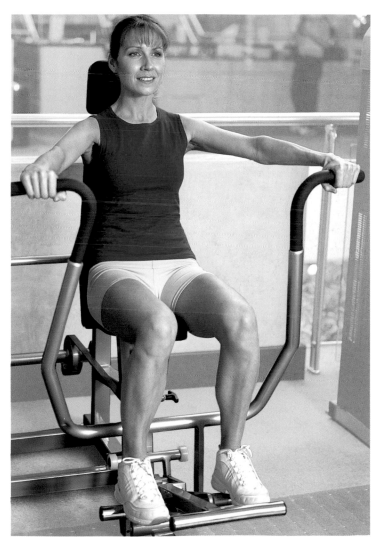

1 To work the pectoralis major, anterior deltoid, and the triceps: sit with your back against the padded back support, with the seat adjusted so that your knees are bent at a right angle. Use the foot bar to bring the handles forwards. Take a wide grip on top of the handle bars. Start with your arms bent at 90 degrees, the elbows positioned just below shoulder level.

2 Exhale and push forwards until your arms are almost straight. Inhale as you slowly bend your elbows to release back.

IN THE GYM: THE PEC DEC

Some pec-dec machines work both the chest and the midback with a simple adjustment of the handles, as here. You can perform the Chest Flye with free weights (*see p104*), and the Reverse Flye with a band (*see p52*) or with free weights (*see p112 and p115*). The machine holds you in proper alignment, which is an advantage for beginners; with free weights you need to stabilize yourself.

CHEST FLYE

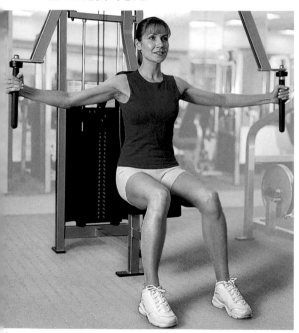

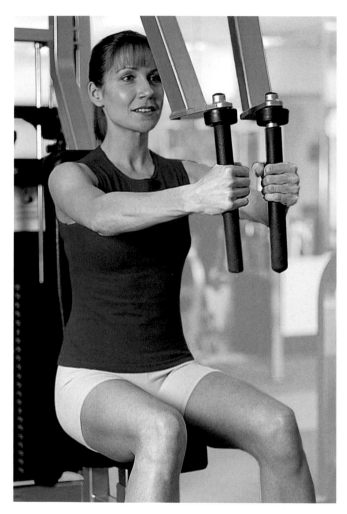

1 Sit tall on the seat, facing forwards, with your lower back and hips pressed firmly into the back support. Your knees should be hip-width apart, directly over your ankles. Position the handles so that your arms are fully extended out to the sides with the elbows slightly rounded. Anchor your shoulder blades by drawing them down and together.

2 Exhale to pull the handles together to the centre of your chest. Pause briefly, then inhale, and release the handles slowly to the start position, taking care not to let your elbows go behind your body.

WEIGHTS & REPETITIONS FOR MACHINE SHOWN

Chest Flye For shaping and toning, set the machine at 14–16kg (30–35lb) and do 12–15 reps. **For bone building**, set the machine at 18–20kg (40–45lb) and do 8–12 reps. **Reverse Flye** For shaping and toning, set the machine at 9–11kg (20–25lb) and do 12–15 reps. **For bone building**, set the machine at 14–16kg (30–35lb) and do 8–12 reps. *Note: Weights on machines vary widely. Be sure to consult with staff at your gym as to how a particular machine works.*

☐ REVERSE FLYE

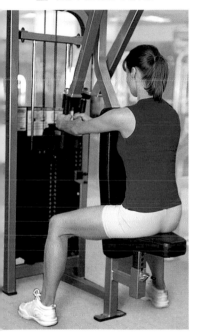

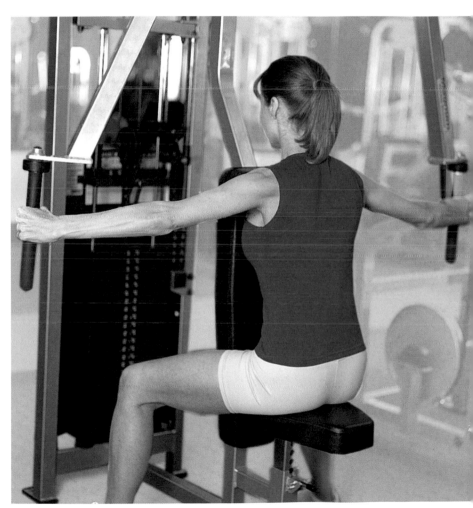

1 This exercise strengthens the muscles of the midback to counteract slouching. Sit tall on the seat, facing into the machine, with your chest against the back support. Position the handles so that your arms are extended in front of your chest. Anchor your shoulder blades.

2 Exhale and pull the handles out to the sides, to the midline of your body only. Pause briefly, then inhale as you slowly release the handles to the start position. Keep your elbows softly bent throughout the movement.

THE SHOULDER: DELTOID

The deltoid sits like an epaulette on top of the shoulder. Although it is one muscle that covers the entire shoulder joint, the deltoid is often referred to by its three aspects, or parts: the anterior (front), medial (middle), and posterior (rear) deltoid. Toning each part of the deltoid gives a beautiful shape to the shoulder and creates a perfect "hanger" for clothing. It can be tricky to work the shoulder area without tensing the neck. I have found the following exercises to be highly effective in targeting each part of the deltoid without strain. Keep the weights light and focus on isolating the muscle.

WEIGHTS & REPETITIONS

Shaping and toning Standing only, use 1–2kg (2–5lb) free weights. For exercises lying, use 0.5–1kg (1–3lb) free weights. Do 12–15 reps per set.

Bone building Standing only, use 4kg (8lb) free weights. For exercises lying, use 2kg (5lb) free weights. Do 8–12 reps per set.

☐ STANDING FRONT RAISE

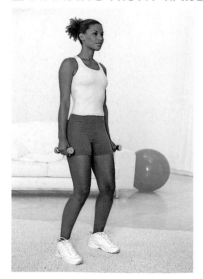

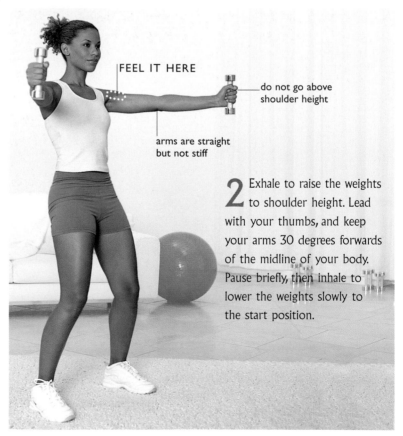

FEEL IT HERE

do not go above shoulder height

arms are straight but not stiff

1 To work the anterior deltoid: stand with your feet parallel, hip-width apart. Hold a free weight in each hand, palms facing in. Brace your shoulder blades by drawing them down and together.

2 Exhale to raise the weights to shoulder height. Lead with your thumbs, and keep your arms 30 degrees forwards of the midline of your body. Pause briefly, then inhale to lower the weights slowly to the start position.

SIDE-LYING LATERAL RAISE

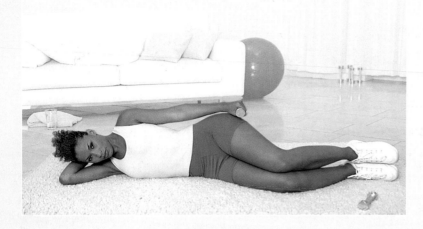

1 To emphasize the medial deltoid: lie on your side on a mat or a well-padded surface. With hips stacked, shoulder to the ceiling, bend both knees 45 degrees forwards of the body. Rest your head on your bent arm, a small pillow, or a folded towel. Hold a free weight at your hip with your palm down, elbow straight. Draw your shoulder blade down.

2 Keeping the palm down, exhale as you lift the weight to shoulder height. Your arm should be straight but not stiff. Pause briefly, then inhale as you lower your arm slowly to the start position.

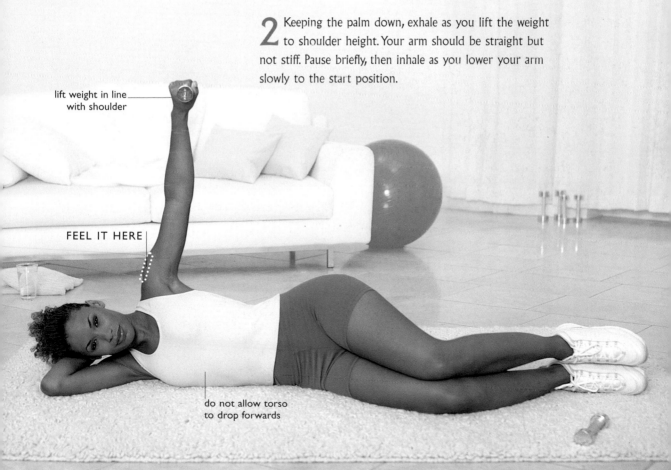

lift weight in line with shoulder

FEEL IT HERE

do not allow torso to drop forwards

SIDE-LYING REVERSE FLYE

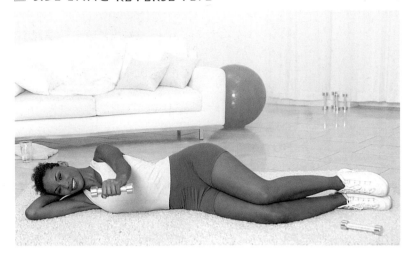

This exercise works the posterior deltoid, which tends to be weak in many women. Strengthening it will help to stabilize the shoulder joint, improve posture, and reduce strain in your back and neck.

1 Lie on your side as before. Hold the free weight out to the front at shoulder level, with your palm down, elbow straight. Draw your shoulder blade down.

2 Exhale as you lift the weight to the midline of your body above your shoulder. Keep your palm facing forwards. Pause briefly, then inhale as you lower your arm slowly to the start position.

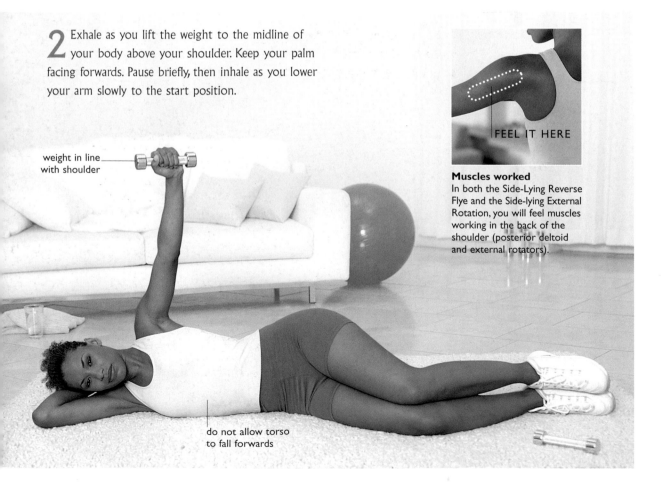

weight in line with shoulder

do not allow torso to fall forwards

FEEL IT HERE

Muscles worked
In both the Side-Lying Reverse Flye and the Side-lying External Rotation, you will feel muscles working in the back of the shoulder (posterior deltoid and external rotators).

SIDE-LYING EXTERNAL ROTATION

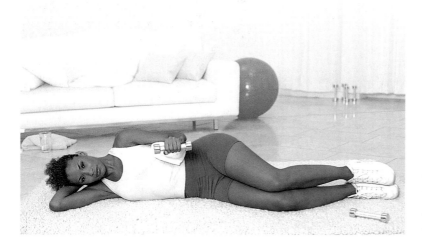

Strengthening the rotator cuff muscles reinforces the shoulder joint to prevent injury (*see also p53*). The towel is critical in this exercise for proper alignment of the arm to the shoulder.

1 Lie on your side as before. Put a folded towel under your upper arm and "pin" it to your side with your elbow. Keep your elbow bent at a right angle and hold the free weight with the palm down.

2 Exhale as you rotate the weight to the ceiling. Pause, then inhale as you slowly return to the start position. Do all your reps, then turn over to your other side and repeat the whole sequence with the other arm, starting with the Side-Lying Lateral Raise on p111.

TRAINER'S TIPS

• **In each exercise,** before you begin moving your arm, brace your shoulder blade by drawing it down and together.
• **Keep the weights** light to isolate the muscle properly.
• **Relax your neck** (a pillow under your neck may help). If you feel any strain, lighten the free weight or do the exercises without a weight.

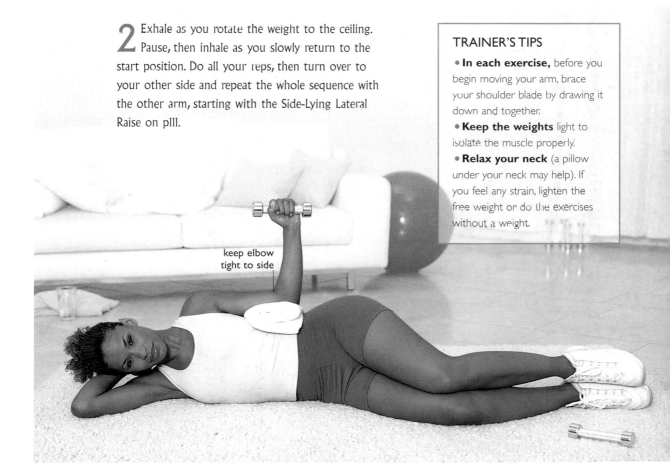

keep elbow tight to side

■ "Ys" AND "Ts" ON BALL

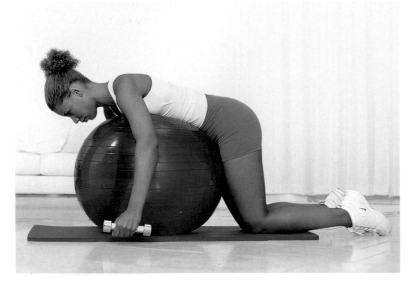

The stability ball creates an unstable base for performing the Front Raise (*p110*) and the Reverse Flye (*p112*). For even more of a challenge, straighten your legs so that your toes are supporting your torso on the ball.

1 The "Y" movement targets the anterior deltoid: kneel on a mat and rest your ribcage on top of the stability ball. Hold a free weight in each hand, palms facing in.

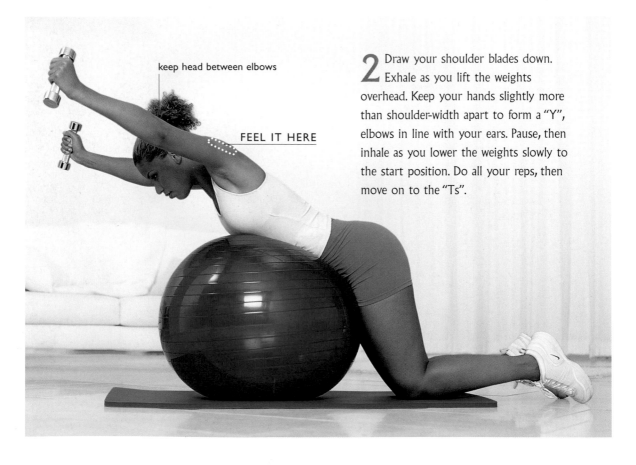

keep head between elbows

FEEL IT HERE

2 Draw your shoulder blades down. Exhale as you lift the weights overhead. Keep your hands slightly more than shoulder-width apart to form a "Y", elbows in line with your ears. Pause, then inhale as you lower the weights slowly to the start position. Do all your reps, then move on to the "Ts".

TRAINER'S TIPS
- **Keep your head** and neck in alignment with your spine.
- **Draw your shoulder blades** together before initiating the movement with the arms.
- **Keep the elbows** soft to avoid stress to the joint.
- **Lift the arms** without momentum, or swinging them as you perform the action.

3 The "Ts" work the posterior deltoid: from the start position, as before, draw your shoulder blades down and together. Exhale as you lift your arms out to the sides, until your elbows are level with your shoulders, forming a "T". Keep your palms down. Pause, then inhale as you lower the weights slowly to the start position.

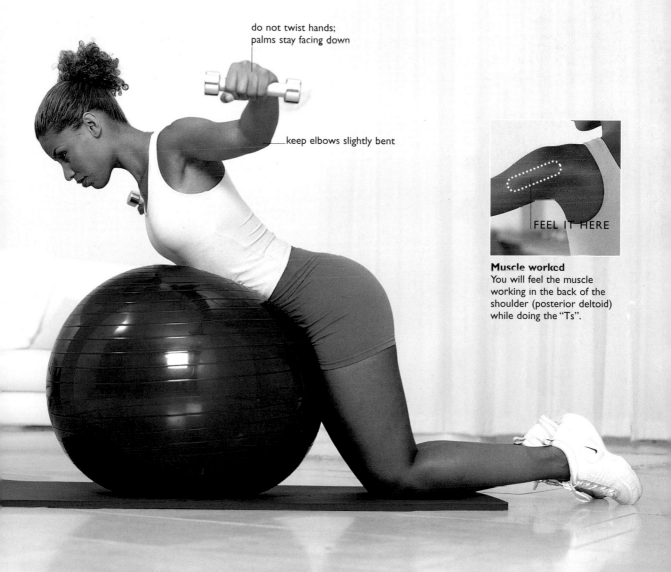

do not twist hands; palms stay facing down

keep elbows slightly bent

FEEL IT HERE

Muscle worked
You will feel the muscle working in the back of the shoulder (posterior deltoid) while doing the "Ts".

THE UPPER ARM: BICEPS

Occasionally a client comes to me for beautiful arms for her wedding dress – her enthusiasm and commitment make the training fun for both of us. Biceps curls will improve the shape of the upper arm noticeably. They will also strengthen the arm for greater ease in day-to-day activities that involve pulling, lifting, and carrying. You'll appreciate the difference the next time you have to carry heavy shopping or your own luggage. If you start swinging your arms or rocking back and forth, the weights are too heavy.

WEIGHTS & REPETITIONS

Shaping and toning 1–2kg (3–5lb) free weights. For Curls, do 12–15 reps on each arm per set; for "21s", do 21 reps per set.

Bone building 4–5kg (8–10lb) free weights. For Curls, do 8–12 reps on each arm per set; for "21s", do 21 reps per set.

☐ ALTERNATING BICEPS CURL

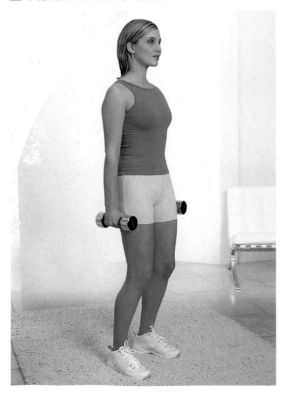

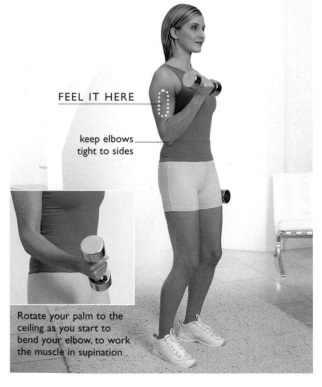

FEEL IT HERE

keep elbows tight to sides

Rotate your palm to the ceiling as you start to bend your elbow, to work the muscle in supination

1 Stand with your feet parallel, hip-width apart, knees soft. Hold a free weight in each hand, with your arms straight at your sides, wrists aligned with the forearm, palms facing in.

2 Exhale and squeeze your upper arm as you bend your right elbow, lifting the weight towards your shoulder. To return, inhale and straighten your forearm fully, maintaining tension in the muscle. Do all your reps, alternating arms.

■ BICEPS "21s"

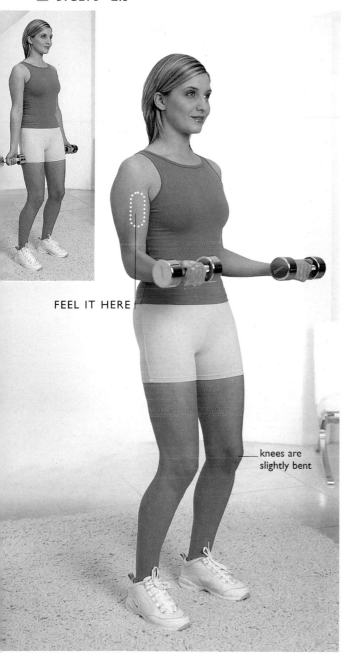

FEEL IT HERE

knees are
slightly bent

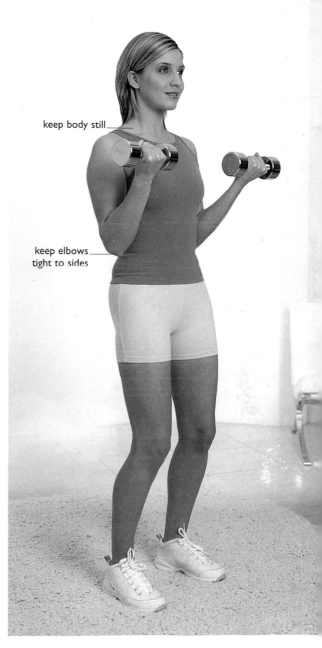

keep body still

keep elbows
tight to sides

1 Stand as before, with your palms facing forwards. To work the lower range of motion, keep your elbows tight to your sides and exhale to lift the free weights as high as your elbows. Inhale and slowly lower them. Do 7 reps.

2 To work the upper range of motion, exhale to raise the weights from the elbow to the shoulder for 7 reps. Then do 7 reps working the full range of motion, raising the weights all the way up and down.

THE UPPER ARM: TRICEPS 1

My clients are always asking me for the best exercises to firm up the back of the upper arm. It is one of the most common trouble spots for many women, so I like to target it with a variety of exercises. This is one of my favourites. We start with a basic version that supports the torso and exercises one arm at a time. The advanced exercise requires stabilization throughout the body, but the bent-over position is not recommended if you have lower-back problems or a spinal condition (it applies too much force to any weakened vertebrae).

WEIGHTS & REPETITIONS

Shaping and toning 1–2kg (3–5lb) free weights. Do 12–15 reps per set (for Triceps Kickback with Support, do 12–15 reps per arm).

Bone building 4kg (8lb) free weights. Do 8–12 reps per set (for Triceps Kickback with Support, do 8–12 reps per arm).

☐ TRICEPS KICKBACK WITH SUPPORT

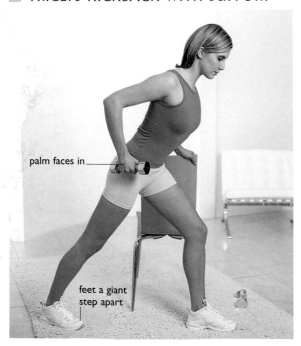

palm faces in

feet a giant step apart

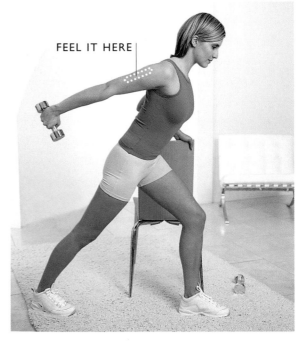

FEEL IT HERE

1 Place your left hand on a chair back for support and take a staggered lunge position, your left, front knee bent over the ankle. Hold a weight in your right hand. Keeping your spine straight, bend forwards from the hip. Bend the right elbow to 90 degrees and raise the upper arm so that it is as parallel to the floor as you can get it.

2 Keeping your abdominal muscles tight, exhale as your extend the forearm behind you so that your arm is straight. Pause and squeeze the back of the upper arm. Inhale to return slowly to the start position, keeping the upper arm stationary. Do all your reps, then turn around to repeat on the left arm.

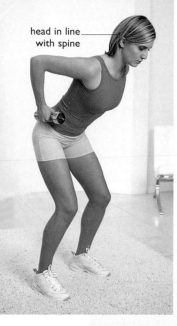

head in line with spine

■ UNSUPPORTED TRICEPS KICKBACK

1 Stand with your feet parallel, hip-width apart, knees bent. Bend forwards from the hip, keeping your spine straight. Holding weights in both hands with the palms facing in, bend your elbows to 90 degrees and raise the upper arms so that they are parallel to the floor.

FEEL IT HERE

maintain natural curve in lower back

2 Keeping your abdominal muscles tight, exhale as you extend your forearms behind you so that your arms are straight but not stiff. Pause and squeeze the backs of the upper arms. Inhale as you slowly return to the start position. Your head should remain in line with your spine throughout the exercise.

THE UPPER ARM: TRICEPS 2

To bare arms with confidence, we can never do too many different exercises to firm and strengthen the triceps, adding muscle tone and shape to the back of the upper arm. For best results, choose two or three different exercises to rotate in your programme (*see also pp118–119 and the Lying Triceps Extension, p105*). These two are "good to go" since you can do them anywhere, one using a portable stretch band, the other relying on your own body weight.

☐ ONE-ARM TRICEPS PUSH-DOWN

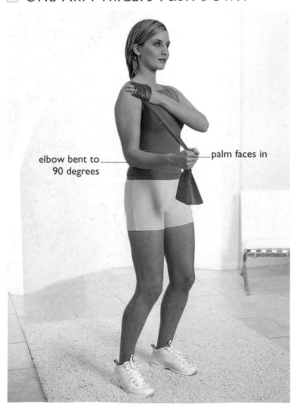

elbow bent to 90 degrees — palm faces in

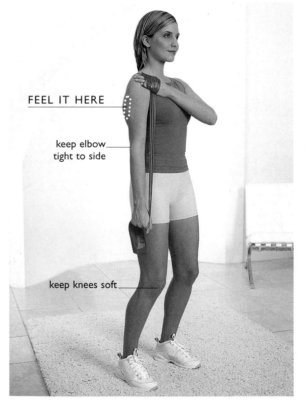

FEEL IT HERE

keep elbow tight to side

keep knees soft

1 Stand with your feet parallel, hip-width apart. To anchor the band, wrap one end around your hand, cross it over your chest, and place it on the opposite shoulder. Hold the band taut with the working arm.

2 Exhale and straighten your arm. Tighten the back of your arm and pause. Inhale to release slowly back to the start position. Do all your reps, keeping tension in the band throughout, then switch arms.

■ SIDE-LYING TRICEPS PRESS-UP

This exercise uses only body weight for resistance, but it's a killer! Start with as many as you can manage, perhaps 3–4 reps per side, and progress as you can to 10–15 reps per side.

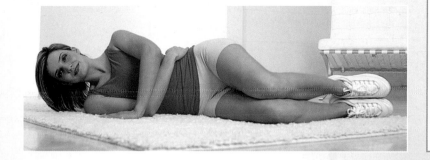

TRAINER'S TIPS

• **Anchor your** shoulder blades by drawing them down and together to keep the chest open.
• **Keep your shoulders** square to the front.
• **Do not twist** through the torso; keep your side to the ceiling.
• **Work your weaker arm** first. If you start with your stronger arm, you will not be able to match the reps on the other side.

1 Lie on your side on a mat or a well-padded surface. Bend your knees so that they are 45 degrees in front of your body. Wrap your bottom arm around your waist. Place your working hand on the floor slightly in front of you with the fingers pointing towards your head, and your elbow bent at a right angle. Your head is raised in line with your spine.

2 Exhale and press through your working arm until it is nearly straight, lifting your torso off the floor. Pause, then inhale as you lower yourself slowly back to the floor. Repeat without resting until you can do no more. Switch sides and repeat.

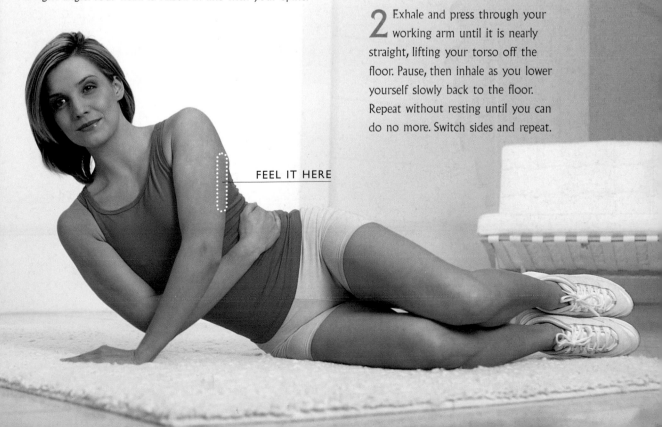

FEEL IT HERE

UPPER BODY STRETCHES

These simple stretches are beneficial for overall well-being, to counteract the physical stressors of our day-to-day activities, and to discharge tension from the neck and shoulders. They can be done either standing or sitting – you can even do them if you are at your desk and you start to feel tight anywhere in your upper body. As you perform each of these stretches, remember to keep your shoulders level and square to the front.

☐ NECK TILT

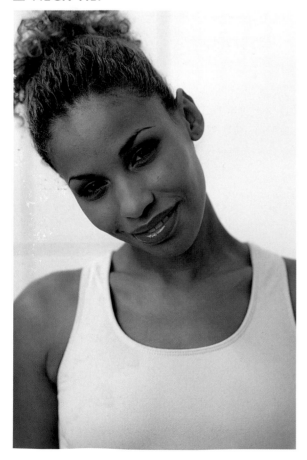

Rest your arms by your sides. Tilt your ear to your shoulder until you feel gentle pulling in the opposite side of the neck. Hold for 5–10 seconds, then switch sides. Repeat 3 times on each side.

☐ CHIN-TO-CHEST STRETCH

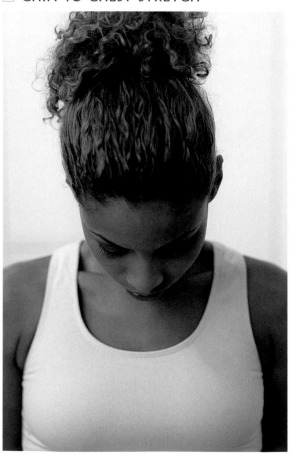

Rest your arms by your sides. Keep your back straight and gently lower your chin towards your chest until you feel the stretch in the back of the neck and the upper back. Hold for 5–10 seconds. Repeat 3 times.

☐ POSTERIOR-DELTOID STRETCH

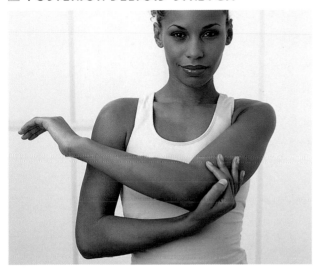

Draw your shoulder blades down and together. Bring one arm in front of your body and gently pull it across your chest with the other hand above the elbow, stretching the back of the shoulder. Hold for 10 seconds on each side.

☐ TRICEPS STRETCH

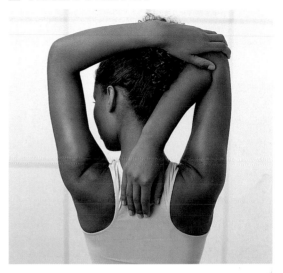

Raise one elbow to the ceiling and reach down your spine with the forearm. Use the other arm to pull back gently on the elbow. Feel the stretch in the back of the upper arm. Hold for 10 seconds on each side.

☐ ANTERIOR-DELTOID STRETCH

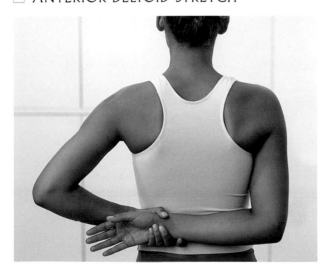

Put one arm behind you and take it by the wrist with your other hand. Gently pull the back arm across the back of your waist until you feel the stretch in the front of the shoulder. Hold for 10 seconds on each side.

☐ BICEPS AND FOREARM STRETCH

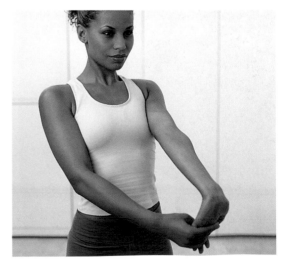

Extend one arm in front of you with the palm up. With the other hand, pull back on the palm. You will feel a stretch all the way up the underside of your arm to the biceps. Hold for 10 seconds on each side.

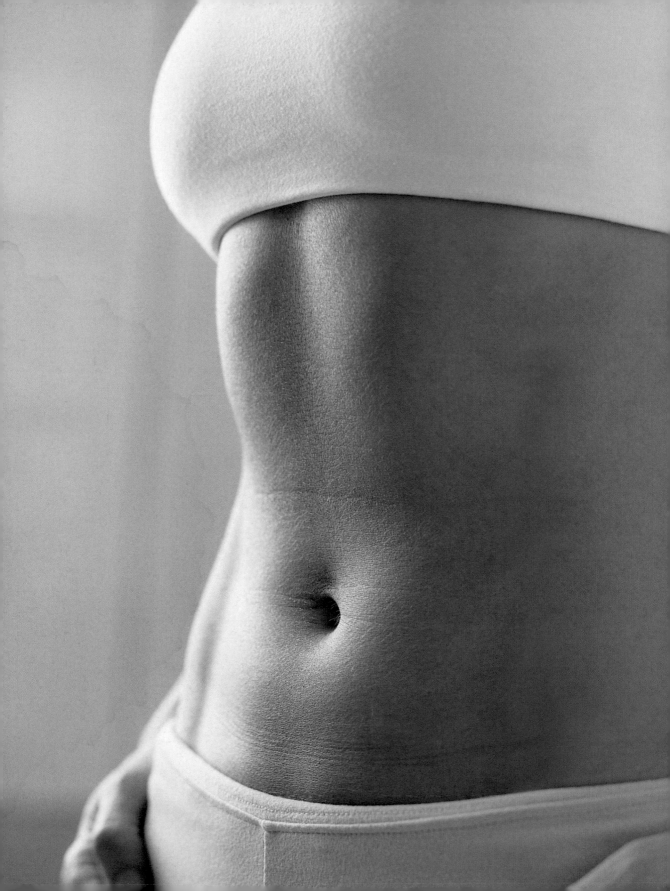

CORE BODY PROGRAMME

In my training sessions, I usually save the exercises for the core body until last, since most of them are done on the floor and can conveniently precede the cooling-down floor stretches. Instead of doing endless crunches, which only work one muscle of the abdomen, you need to work all the abdominal muscles in a variety of exercises for a flatter belly and a trimmer waist. Doing the back exercises balances out your core-body workout by giving you stronger support for the spine and improving your posture. Both the abdominals and the back muscles work together in the plank exercises (*pp138–141*) to improve core stabilization.

"Joan's outstanding knowledge, attentiveness, and caring make her the best trainer I have ever had. She has inspired me to become a trainer myself, and I look forward to her continued guidance both as a client and as a trainer."
Liliane K.

PROGRAMMES AT A GLANCE

Work through the programmes below, starting with Level 1 and building up to Level 3. Alternatively, pick at least one exercise for the rectus abdominis and one for the transversus abdominis to complete your own whole-body programme of 8–10 exercises. If you have more time, add exercises for the obliques and the spinal extensors.

LEVEL 1 (BEGINNER)

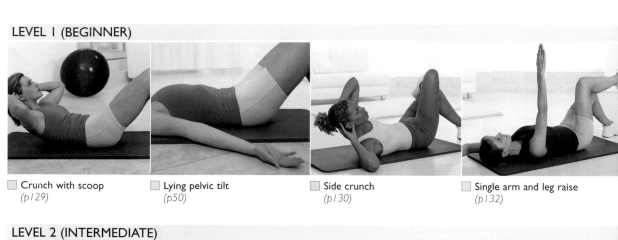

■ Crunch with scoop *(p129)*　　■ Lying pelvic tilt *(p50)*　　■ Side crunch *(p130)*　　■ Single arm and leg raise *(p132)*

LEVEL 2 (INTERMEDIATE)

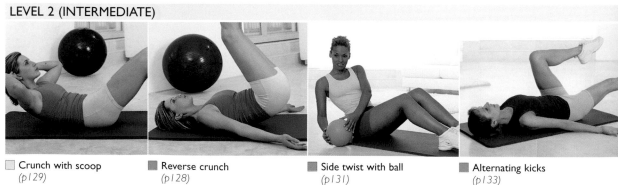

■ Crunch with scoop *(p129)*　　■ Reverse crunch *(p128)*　　■ Side twist with ball *(p131)*　　■ Alternating kicks *(p133)*

LEVEL 3 (ADVANCED)

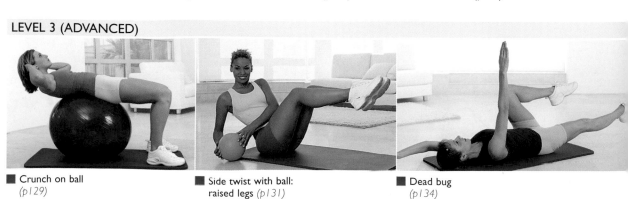

■ Crunch on ball *(p129)*　　■ Side twist with ball: raised legs *(p131)*　　■ Dead bug *(p134)*

TRAINING GUIDELINES

- Remember to warm up (pp32–37) before you start and to stretch out (pp146–149) after working the muscles.
- Use proper body alignment and good form.
- Start gently and avoid pain.
- Gradually increase the intensity.

- Use the colour code to guide you in your choice of exercise:

▢ Beginner: suitable for most people

▨ Intermediate: requires more strength and coordination

▉ Advanced: challenges strength and balance

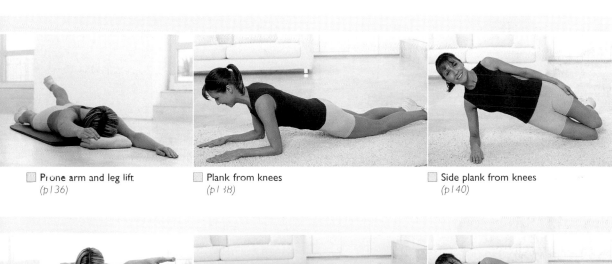

▢ Prone arm and leg lift
(p136)

▢ Plank from knees
(p138)

▢ Side plank from knees
(p140)

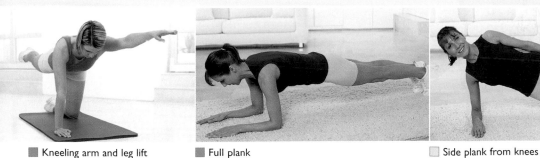

▨ Kneeling arm and leg lift
(p137)

▨ Full plank
(p139)

▢ Side plank from knees
(p140)

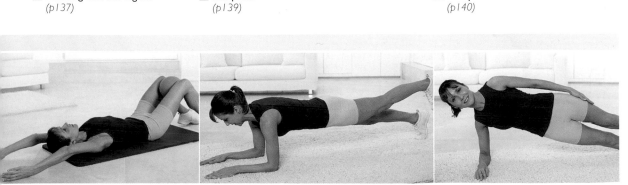

▉ Ball transfer
(p135)

▉ One-legged plank
(p139)

▉ Side plank from feet
(p141)

THE ABS: RECTUS ABDOMINIS

The rectus abdominis is best known as the coveted "six-pack" muscle, which describes the sections that develop when this muscle is toned. It is the most superficial muscle of the abdomen, running from the sternum to the pubic bone. It functions to flex the spine and stabilize the pelvis as you walk. If it is weak, it can lead to an increased arch in the lower back known as a hollow back.

REPETITIONS

Do 15–20 reps per set.

■ REVERSE CRUNCH

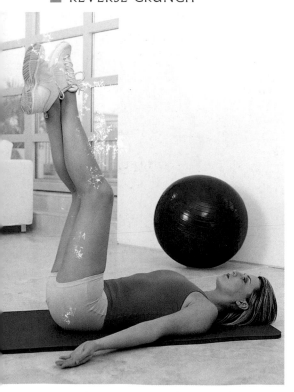

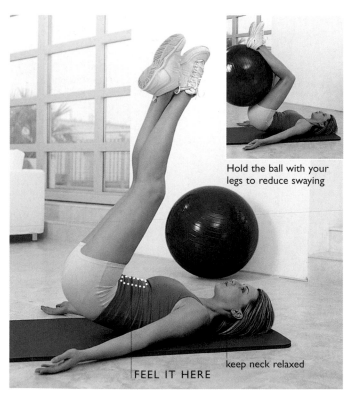

Hold the ball with your legs to reduce swaying

FEEL IT HERE

keep neck relaxed

1 Lie on your back on the mat with your legs raised to the ceiling, your knees over your hips, and your ankles crossed. Relax your arms by your sides with the palms up to keep the shoulders open and decrease any assistance from the arms.

2 Exhale, pulling the belly button towards the spine, and lift your hips off the floor, drawing the pelvis towards the ribcage. Inhale, and with a slow, controlled movement, lower your hips to the floor. Be careful not to use momentum or to swing the legs. Alternatively, hold the stability ball behind your legs to prevent them from swinging.

CRUNCH WITH SCOOP

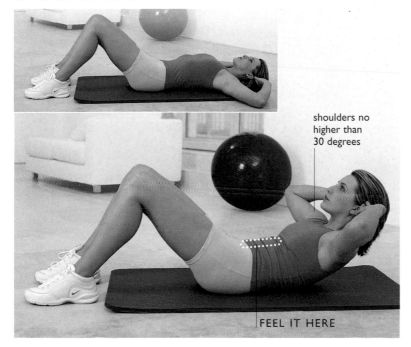

shoulders no
higher than
30 degrees

FEEL IT HERE

Lie on your back on the mat with your knees bent at 90 degrees, feet flat on the floor. To avoid pulling on the neck, place your fingertips behind your ears, hands unclasped, elbows wide. Exhale, scooping out the abdomen, belly button to spine, as you lift the shoulders no more than 30 degrees off the floor (do not go into a full sit-up). Draw the ribs towards the pelvis. Keep your chin up, as if you were holding an orange under it. Pause at the top, then inhale, and slowly lower your shoulders (but not your head) to the floor.

CRUNCH ON BALL

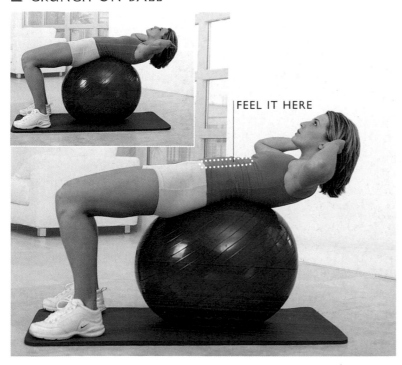

FEEL IT HERE

Recent studies have found this advanced variation to be the most effective at targeting the rectus (followed by the crunch above).

Position yourself on the stability ball, knees bent at 90 degrees, feet hip-width apart. Your lower and mid-back should be supported, upper back and shoulders slightly below the top of ball. Place your fingertips behind your ears, elbows wide. Keep your chin up. Exhale and contract the abs, lifting the shoulders up, lower back pressed firmly against the ball. Pause at the top, then inhale, and slowly return to the start position without releasing the abs.

THE WAIST: OBLIQUES

Even my thinnest clients ask me for ways to trim the waist. Twisting exercises train the internal and external obliques of the abdomen, toning the muscles that shape the sides of the waist and providing the power to twist and turn the torso as well as to keep it erect. The most effective exercises for the obliques work your body at an angle, but avoid them if you have a spinal condition.

REPETITIONS

Do 15–20 reps on each side per set.

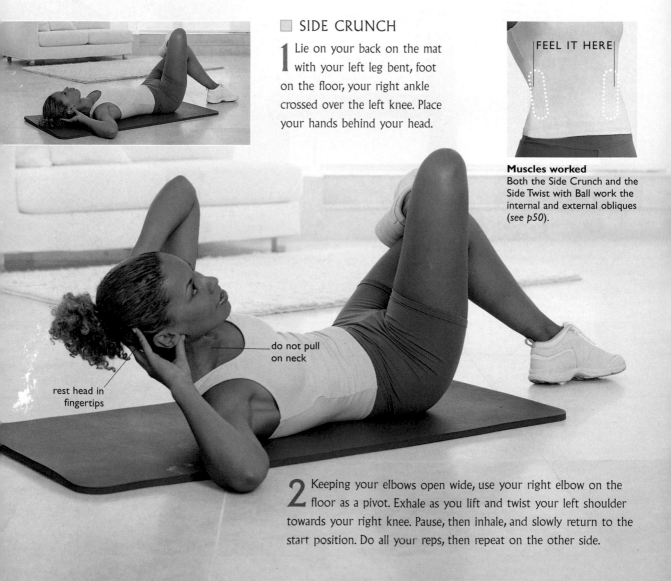

☐ SIDE CRUNCH

1 Lie on your back on the mat with your left leg bent, foot on the floor, your right ankle crossed over the left knee. Place your hands behind your head.

FEEL IT HERE

Muscles worked
Both the Side Crunch and the Side Twist with Ball work the internal and external obliques (see p50).

do not pull on neck

rest head in fingertips

2 Keeping your elbows open wide, use your right elbow on the floor as a pivot. Exhale as you lift and twist your left shoulder towards your right knee. Pause, then inhale, and slowly return to the start position. Do all your reps, then repeat on the other side.

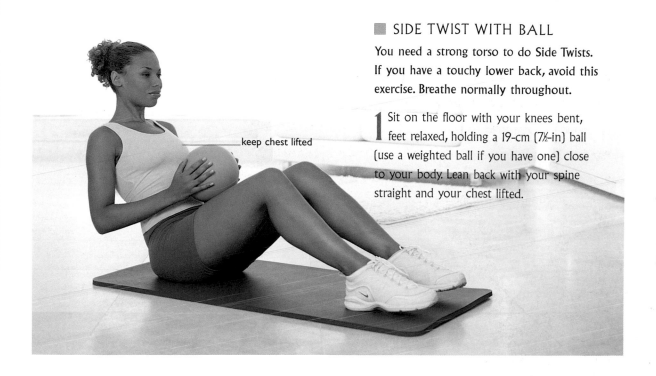

keep chest lifted

■ SIDE TWIST WITH BALL

You need a strong torso to do Side Twists. If you have a touchy lower back, avoid this exercise. Breathe normally throughout.

1 Sit on the floor with your knees bent, feet relaxed, holding a 19-cm (7½-in) ball (use a weighted ball if you have one) close to your body. Lean back with your spine straight and your chest lifted.

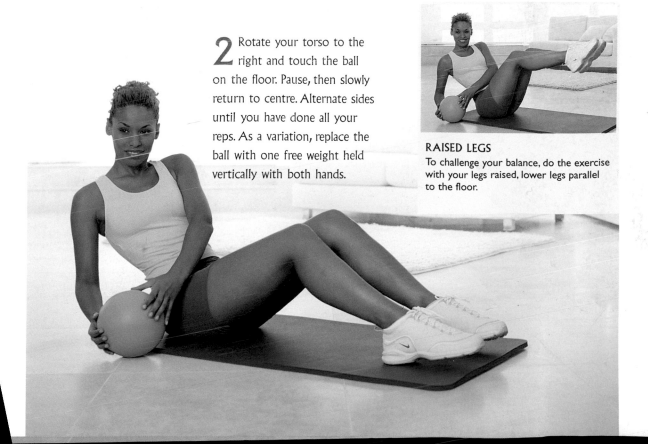

2 Rotate your torso to the right and touch the ball on the floor. Pause, then slowly return to centre. Alternate sides until you have done all your reps. As a variation, replace the ball with one free weight held vertically with both hands.

RAISED LEGS
To challenge your balance, do the exercise with your legs raised, lower legs parallel to the floor.

CORE STABILIZATION

The Plank is a simple move that trains the abdominals and spinal extensors as they work to maintain the raised position. You benefit from improved core strength, tighter abdominals, and a stronger back, all of which create better posture. Although the Full Plank is an advanced exercise, you can build up to it in stages. Concentrate on tightening the muscles of your abdomen, back, buttocks, and legs – and remember to breathe!

REPETITIONS

For Planks on these pages, do once and hold for 10 seconds, progressing to 30 seconds. For the Side Planks (pp140–141), start with holding for 10 seconds and progress to holding for 30 seconds.

☐ PLANK FROM KNEES

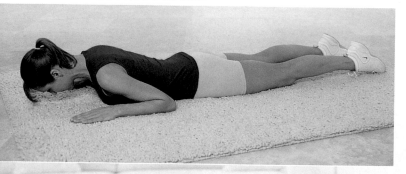

1 Lie face down on a mat or a well-padded surface with your arms bent, elbows close to your sides, palms down. Tighten the abdomen, creating an arch under your stomach.

2 Keeping the abdomen lifted, slide the elbows forwards directly under your shoulders, and lift the hips off the floor, creating a straight line from knee to shoulder. Keep the shoulder blades wide and apart, the spine straight with neutral alignment.

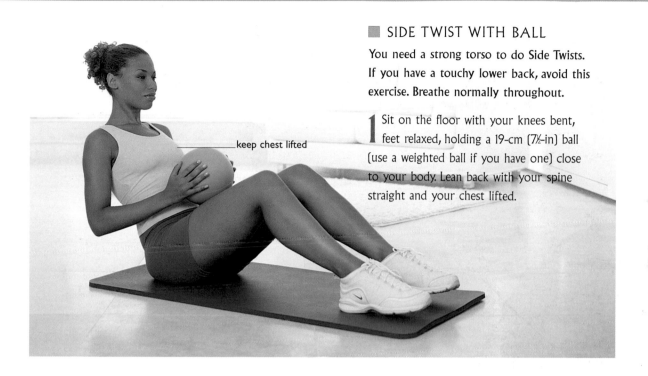

keep chest lifted

■ SIDE TWIST WITH BALL

You need a strong torso to do Side Twists. If you have a touchy lower back, avoid this exercise. Breathe normally throughout.

1 Sit on the floor with your knees bent, feet relaxed, holding a 19-cm (7½-in) ball (use a weighted ball if you have one) close to your body. Lean back with your spine straight and your chest lifted.

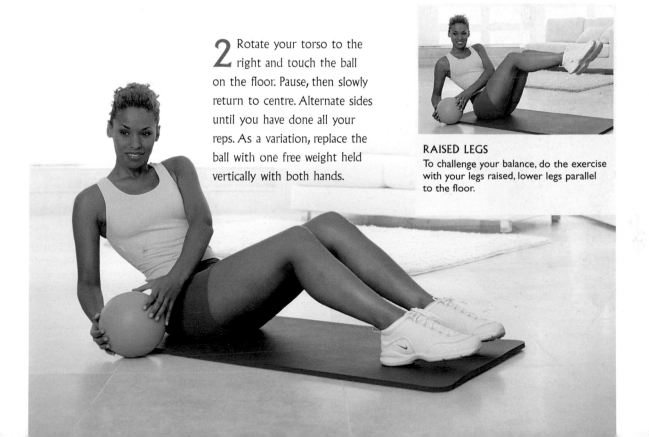

2 Rotate your torso to the right and touch the ball on the floor. Pause, then slowly return to centre. Alternate sides until you have done all your reps. As a variation, replace the ball with one free weight held vertically with both hands.

RAISED LEGS

To challenge your balance, do the exercise with your legs raised, lower legs parallel to the floor.

THE DEEP ABDOMINALS

When it is toned, the transversus abdominis (*see p50*) acts as a natural girdle, flattening the abdomen and supporting the lower back. Here, it is required to stabilize the pelvis against the changing resistance of your arm and leg movements. If you have a spinal condition, these exercises provide an excellent alternative to more traditional abdominal exercises, such as crunches, which round the upper back in spinal flexion and can place stress on the vertebrae.

REPETITIONS

To start, do 5–10 reps on each side per set. Progress to 10 reps on each side per set. In Alternating Kicks (p133) and Dead Bug (p134), hold the extended position for up to 10 seconds.

☐ SINGLE ARM AND LEG RAISE

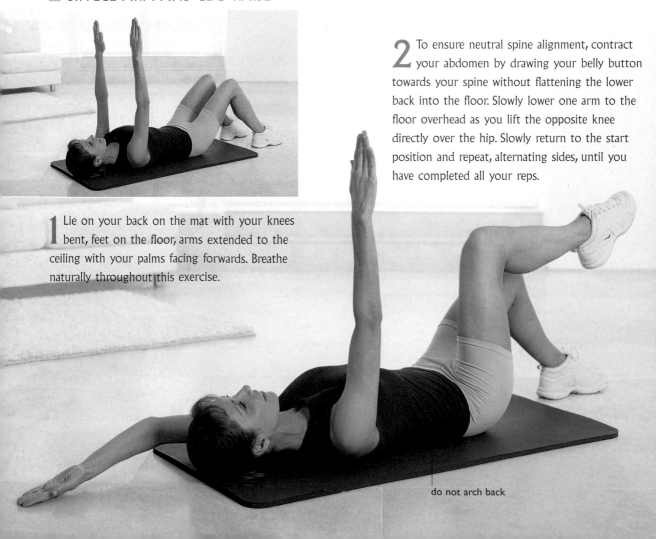

2 To ensure neutral spine alignment, contract your abdomen by drawing your belly button towards your spine without flattening the lower back into the floor. Slowly lower one arm to the floor overhead as you lift the opposite knee directly over the hip. Slowly return to the start position and repeat, alternating sides, until you have completed all your reps.

1 Lie on your back on the mat with your knees bent, feet on the floor, arms extended to the ceiling with your palms facing forwards. Breathe naturally throughout this exercise.

do not arch back

ALTERNATING KICKS

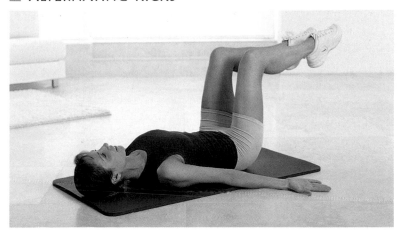

When you can maintain neutral spine alignment in the previous exercise, move on to Alternating Kicks. Breathe naturally throughout.

1 Lie on your back on the mat with your hips and knees bent at 90 degrees. With your arms at your sides, press the backs of your hands into the floor to stabilize your shoulder blades.

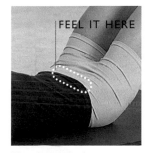

FEEL IT HERE

Muscle worked
Both Single Arm and Leg Raise and Alternating Kicks exercise the transversus abdominis (see p50).

2 With your lower back in neutral spine alignment, abdomen contracted, slowly straighten your right leg, lowering it as close to the floor as possible without arching your back, and bring your left knee in closer to your chest. Pause, then slowly return to the start position and repeat, alternating legs, until you have completed all your reps.

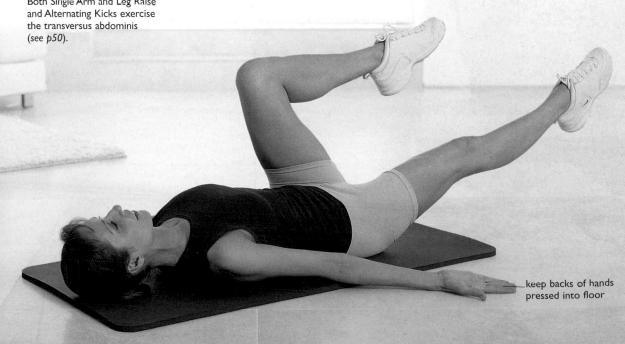

keep backs of hands pressed into floor

■ DEAD BUG

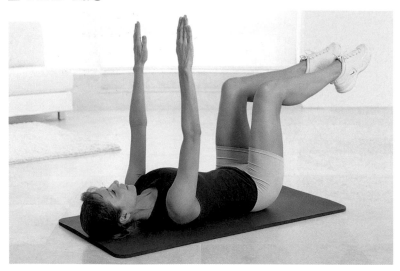

Both Dead Bug and Ball Transfer are often recommended by physical therapists for lower-back conditions. If you have a problem in this area, do these exercises with your lower back pressed to the floor. Breathe naturally throughout.

1 Lie on your back on the mat with your hips and knees bent at 90 degrees, feet in the air. Extend your arms to the ceiling, hands directly over your shoulders, your palms facing forwards.

2 Contract your abdominals by drawing your belly button towards your spine. Lower your left arm overhead and straighten your right leg, lowering it as close to the floor as possible without arching your back. Bring your left, bent knee in closer to your chest. Return to the start position and repeat, alternating sides, until you have completed all your reps.

FEEL IT HERE

Muscle worked
Both Dead Bug and Ball Transfer work the transversus abdominis (see p50).

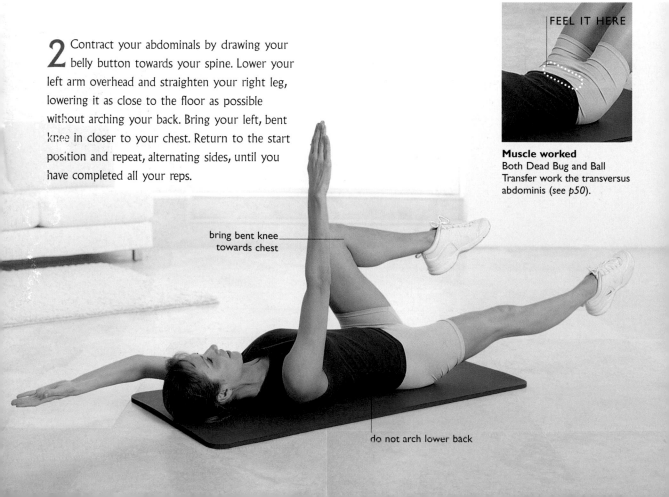

bring bent knee towards chest

do not arch lower back

■ BALL TRANSFER

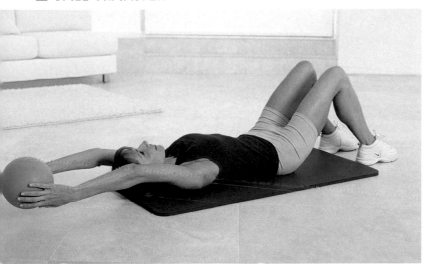

Try this exercise first holding a pillow or a small, unweighted ball. A weighted ball (*see p23*) adds resistance to the exercise. Breathe naturally throughout.

1 Lie on your back on the mat, knees bent, feet flat on the floor. Hold a 19-cm (7½-in) ball overhead with your arms extended and in line with your ears.

2 Contract your abdominals. Keeping your head and shoulders on the floor, raise your arms, and draw your knees up and place the ball between your knees. Lower your arms and feet towards the floor without arching your back. Tap the floor lightly with your hands and toes, but do not rest them, then lift your arms and draw up your knees again to grasp the ball, and return to the start position. (This is 1 rep.) Straightening the legs increases the level of difficulty.

From the second position, with the ball between your knees, raise your arms and legs again to transfer the ball to your hands. Return to the start position.

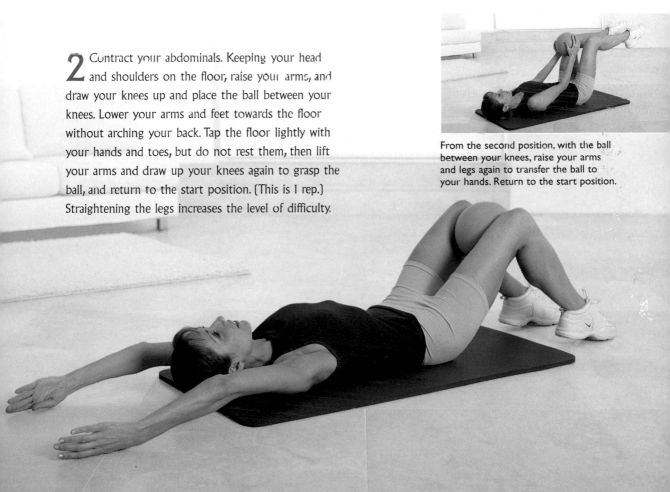

THE BACK: SPINAL EXTENSORS

These exercises strengthen the muscles that support the length of the spine – the spinal extensors – to create stability and help prevent pain in the lower back. Do not do these exercises if you have lower back pain already. They may place too much load on your spine. Wait until you are pain-free, and begin by lifting one leg at a time, then each arm, working around the body. Progress to lifting the opposite arm and leg simultaneously. Breathe naturally throughout.

REPETITIONS

Do 5–10 reps on each side, alternating sides, per set. Progress to 10 reps on each side, alternating sides, holding the extended position for up to 10 seconds.

☐ PRONE ARM AND LEG LIFT

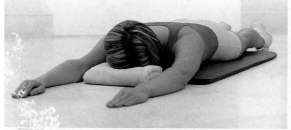

1 Lie face down on the mat with your forehead resting on a folded towel to ensure proper alignment of your head and neck. Extend your arms with the palms down. Lengthen through the torso, reaching the top of your head forwards, and contract your abdominals.

2 Keeping your forehead down, lift one arm and the opposite leg 8–15cm (3–6in) off the floor. Hold for 1 second, then slowly lower your limbs. Repeat on the other side and continue, alternating sides, until you have completed all your reps.

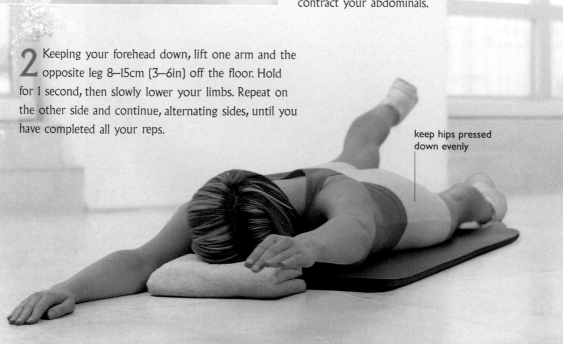

keep hips pressed down evenly

KNEELING ARM AND LEG LIFT

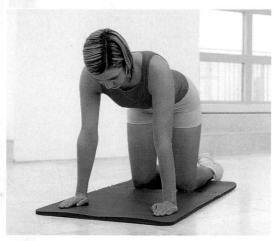

TRAINER'S TIPS

• **Reach forwards** as far as you can with your raised arm while you reach backwards as far as you can with your raised leg.

• **Scoop out your abdominals**, belly button to spine, throughout the movement to prevent your back from arching.

• **Think "nose down"** to keep your head and neck aligned with your spine.

• **Don't twist your torso.** Your shoulders and hips should be square to the floor.

1 Kneel on the mat with your hands under your shoulders and your knees under your hips, your head and neck in alignment with your spine.

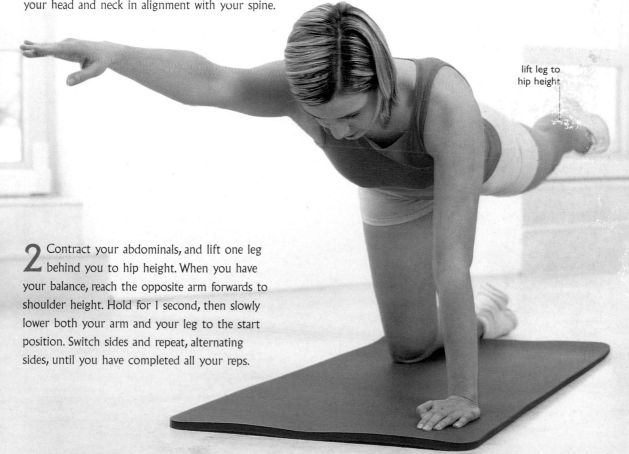

lift leg to hip height

2 Contract your abdominals, and lift one leg behind you to hip height. When you have your balance, reach the opposite arm forwards to shoulder height. Hold for 1 second, then slowly lower both your arm and your leg to the start position. Switch sides and repeat, alternating sides, until you have completed all your reps.

CORE STABILIZATION

The Plank is a simple move that trains the abdominals and spinal extensors as they work to maintain the raised position. You benefit from improved core strength, tighter abdominals, and a stronger back, all of which create better posture. Although the Full Plank is an advanced exercise, you can build up to it in stages. Concentrate on tightening the muscles of your abdomen, back, buttocks, and legs – and remember to breathe!

☐ PLANK FROM KNEES

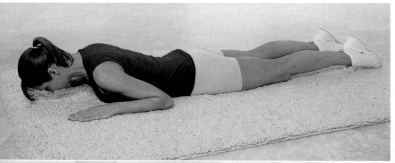

1 Lie face down on a mat or a well-padded surface with your arms bent, elbows close to your sides, palms down. Tighten the abdomen, creating an arch under your stomach.

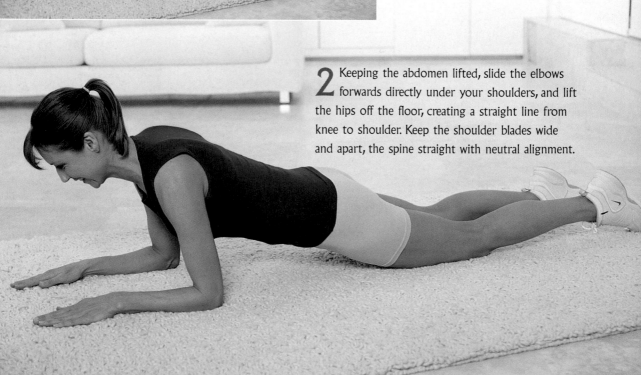

2 Keeping the abdomen lifted, slide the elbows forwards directly under your shoulders, and lift the hips off the floor, creating a straight line from knee to shoulder. Keep the shoulder blades wide and apart, the spine straight with neutral alignment.

■ FULL PLANK

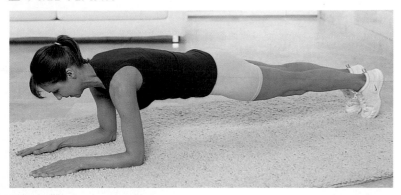

Start as before. Lift up onto your toes, straightening your legs. Draw the shoulder blades down, pressing the forearms into the floor. Maintain length in your neck and a straight line from your shoulders to your ankles.

■ ONE-LEGGED PLANK

After you can hold the Full Plank for 30 seconds, advance by performing it with first one leg lifted in the air and then the other, holding for up to 30 seconds on each leg.

□ SIDE PLANK FROM KNEES

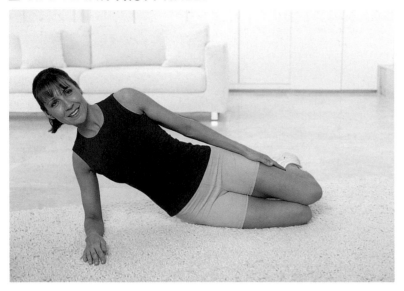

This movement challenges your abdominals in core stabilization and trains the obliques without curving or twisting the spine.

1 Lie on your side propped up on your forearm with your legs bent behind you. Make sure that your supporting elbow is under your shoulder and in line with your hips and knees. Rest your top arm along your side.

2 Contract your abdominals and exhale as you push up on the supporting elbow, lifting your hips off the ground. Keep your ribcage lifted and your shoulder down. Hold for 10–30 seconds, breathing naturally, or repeat 5–10 times. Repeat on the other side.

SUPPORTED SIDE PLANK
While you are learning this exercise, use your top hand on the floor for support.

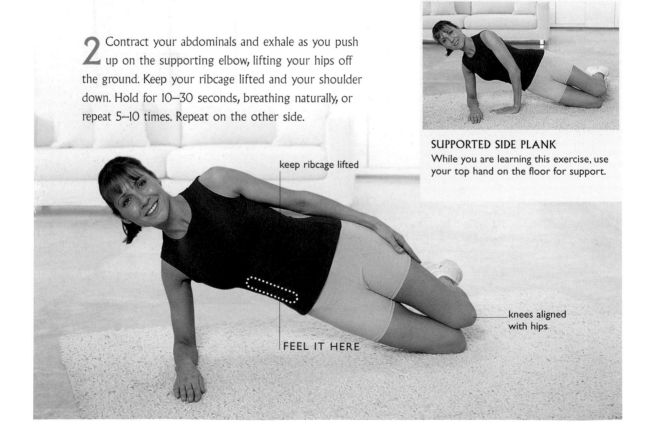

keep ribcage lifted

FEEL IT HERE

knees aligned with hips

■ SIDE PLANK FROM FEET

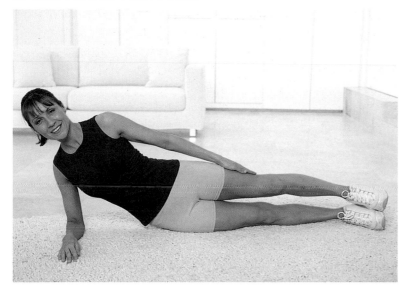

This advanced variation requires you to stabilize throughout the full length of your body.

1 Lie on your side propped up on your elbow with your legs extended, one foot stacked directly on top of the other. Make sure that your supporting elbow is under your shoulder and in line with your hips and feet. Rest your top arm along your side.

2 Contract your abdominals and exhale as you push up on your elbow, lifting your hips off the ground. Your torso should form a straight line with your head and your legs. Hold for 10–30 seconds, breathing naturally, or repeat 5–10 times. Repeat on the other side.

TRAINER'S TIPS

• **Plant your** supporting elbow directly under your shoulder.
• **Line your elbow** up with your hips and your feet so that your body forms a straight line.
• **Keep the ribcage** lifted and the shoulder blades down.

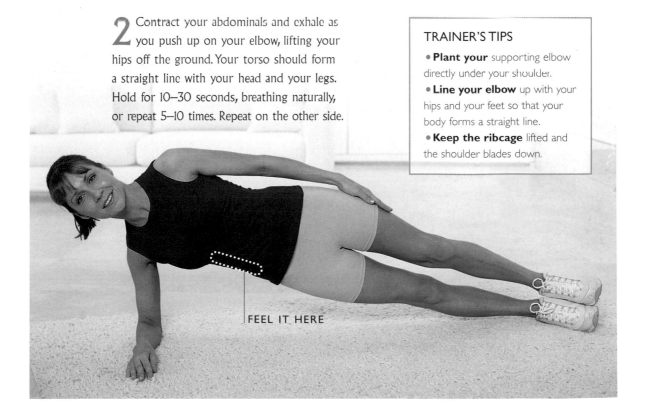

FEEL IT HERE

STRENGTHENING THE WRISTS

Strong wrists improve athletic performance, especially in racket sports and golf. Moreover, it is important to maintain strength in your hands and wrists to perform your daily activities with ease, whether they include computer work, housework, or simple tasks such as being able to open a jar or lift a full tea kettle. In later life, should you stumble, you will be able to break a fall with less risk of fracturing your wrist.

WEIGHTS & REPETITIONS

Shaping and toning 0.5–1kg (1–3lb) free weight. Do 12–15 reps on each hand per set.

Bone building 2–4kg (5–8lb) free weight. Do 8–12 reps on each hand per set.

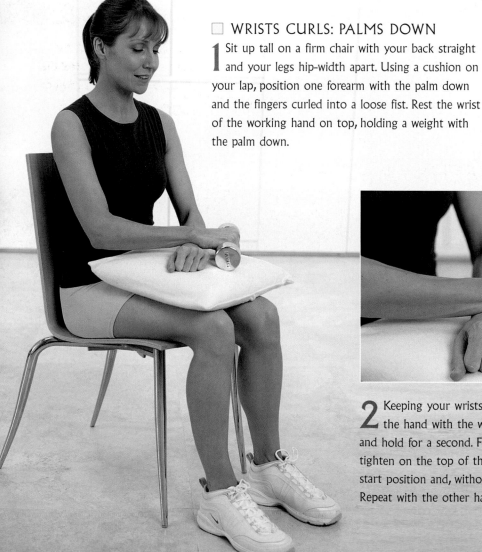

☐ WRISTS CURLS: PALMS DOWN

1 Sit up tall on a firm chair with your back straight and your legs hip-width apart. Using a cushion on your lap, position one forearm with the palm down and the fingers curled into a loose fist. Rest the wrist of the working hand on top, holding a weight with the palm down.

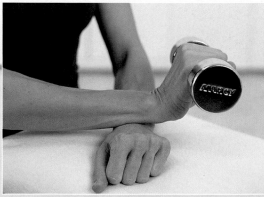

2 Keeping your wrists in contact, lift the back of the hand with the weight towards the ceiling and hold for a second. Feel the muscle tense or tighten on the top of the forearm. Return to the start position and, without resting, do all your reps. Repeat with the other hand.

☐ WRIST CURLS: PALMS UP

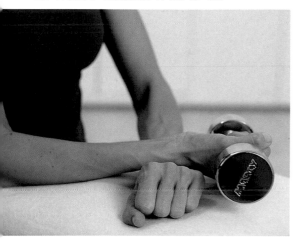

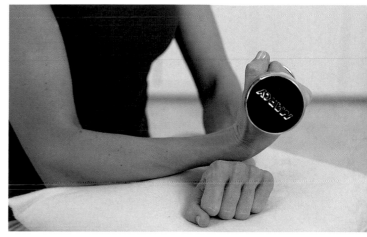

1 Using a cushion on your lap, position one forearm with the palm down and the fingers curled into a loose fist. Rest the back of the working hand on top, holding a weight with the palm up.

2 Keeping your wrists in contact, curl the hand with the weight towards the ceiling and hold for a second. Feel the muscle tense or tighten on the underside of the wrist. Return to the start position and, without resting, do all your reps. Repeat with the other hand.

☐ WRIST CURLS: PRONATION AND SUPINATION

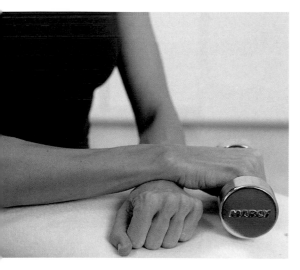

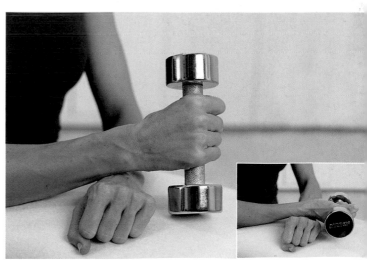

1 Position one forearm with the palm down and the fingers curled into a loose fist as before. Place the other hand palm down holding a weight.

2 Keeping the elbow of the working arm stable, rotate the forearm until the palm is facing up. Turn the forearm back to the start position and, without resting, do all your reps. Repeat with the other hand.

STRENGTHENING THE ANKLES

Of all the muscles in the body, the earliest declines in muscle strength occur around age 40 in the muscles of the lower leg. The changes happen imperceptibly over the decades, and have a dramatic impact on walking ability in the later years. These simple exercises strengthen the ankles to keep you walking in high heels and moving with confidence as you play sports.

> **WEIGHTS & REPETITIONS**
>
> **Shaping and toning** Light to medium band. Do 12–15 reps per set.
>
> **Bone building** Heavy band. Do 8–12 reps per set.

☐ TOE LIFTS

1 Tie the band around a secure object, like the leg of a couch. Sit up tall with the right leg extended in front of you and the band looped around your forefoot. Put a little tension in the band. This is the start position for all three exercises.

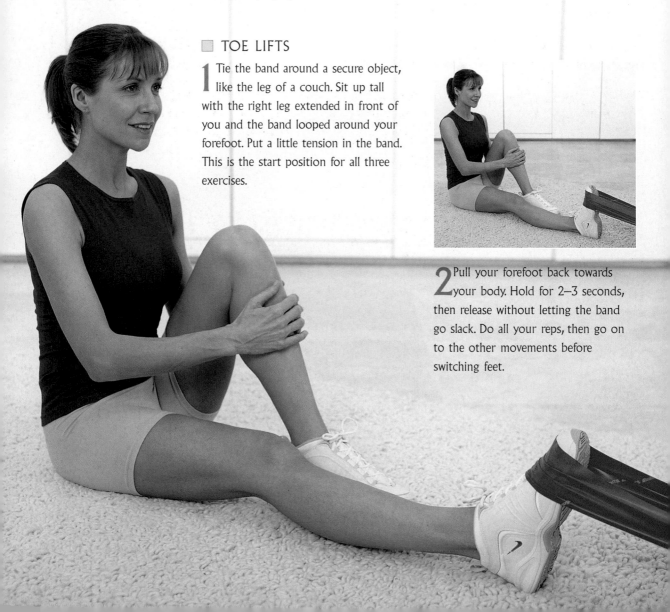

2 Pull your forefoot back towards your body. Hold for 2–3 seconds, then release without letting the band go slack. Do all your reps, then go on to the other movements before switching feet.

INNER-SOLE TWIST

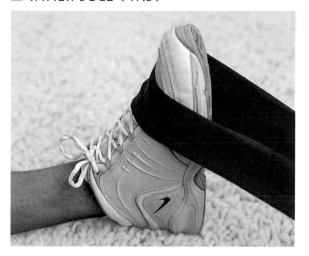

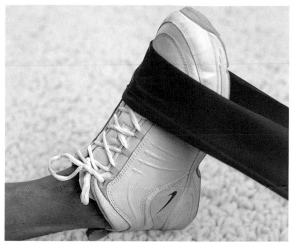

1 From the start position on the opposite page, reposition your right foot about 5–7.5cm (2–3in) to the left so that the band pulls against the inner edge of the forefoot.

2 Keeping your heel on the floor, twist the sole of your right foot inwards and upwards. Hold for 2–3 seconds and repeat. Only the foot should move.

OUTER-SOLE TWIST

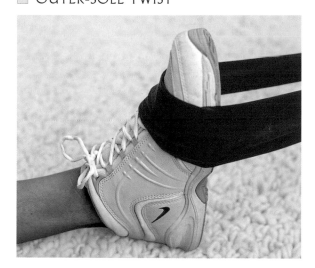

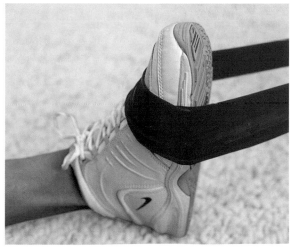

1 From the start position on the opposite page, reposition your right foot about 5–7.5cm (2–3in) to the right so that the band pulls against the outer edge of the forefoot.

2 Keeping your heel on the floor, twist the sole of your foot outwards and upwards. Hold for 2–3 seconds and repeat. Only your foot should move. When you have completed all your reps, do the entire sequence on the left foot.

COOLING DOWN STRETCHES

There is a certain choreography to a fitness training session in the way one exercise flows to the next. I prefer to start with the more intense standing exercises, and gradually work down to the floor, usually ending the session with abdominal work. Along the way, I stretch the upper body muscles we have used, so that by the time we get to the cool-down stretches, we can focus on full-body stretches that release tension from the major muscle groups.

☐ FULL-BODY STRETCH

Lie on your back on the mat. Take a deep breath in and stretch your arms and legs out as far as you can. Exhale, and let your muscles go limp. Repeat 3 times: "Inhale and reach, exhale and release."

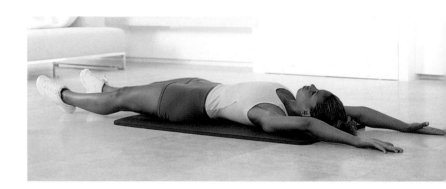

☐ THE BRIDGE

Lie on your back with your knees bent, hands by your sides. Start at the base of your spine and peel your back off the floor, one vertebra at a time, until your body is in a straight line from your knees to your shoulders. As you release down, pay special attention to rolling through the curve in the lower back, and touching down one vertebra at a time.

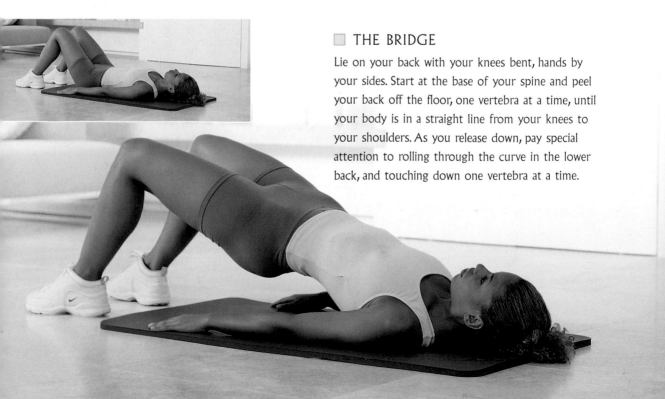

▢ LOWER-BACK STRETCH

Lie on your back and bring both knees up over your chest. Separate your legs and place your hands underneath the thighs. Exhale as you draw your knees up towards your shoulders and your hips curl up slightly from the floor. Inhale and release. Repeat 3 times.

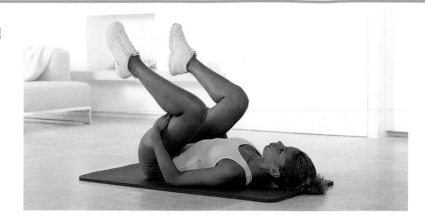

▢ HAMSTRING STRETCH

Lie on your back with your knees bent. Keep one knee bent with the foot on the floor and raise the other leg to the ceiling. Hold the extended leg with both hands behind the thigh and pull it towards you gently, keeping the knee straight. Hold for 20–30 seconds, then repeat with the other leg.

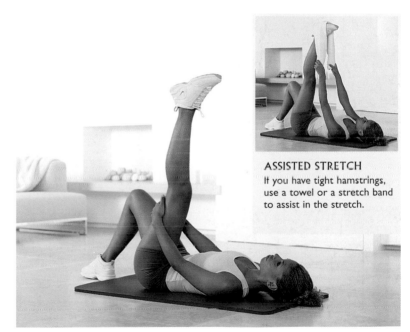

ASSISTED STRETCH
If you have tight hamstrings, use a towel or a stretch band to assist in the stretch.

▢ FOOT CIRCLES

From the Hamstring Stretch above, bend one knee with the foot in the air and circle the ankle 4 times in each direction. Repeat with the other foot.

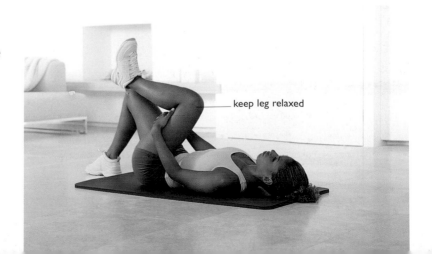

keep leg relaxed

☐ SPINAL TWIST

Lie on your back on the mat with both knees bent and your feet on the floor. Reach your arms out in line with your shoulders, palms down. Drop your knees to one side and turn your head in the opposite direction. Hold for 20–30 seconds and then change sides, being careful to pull your lower back to the floor before you twist to the opposite side.

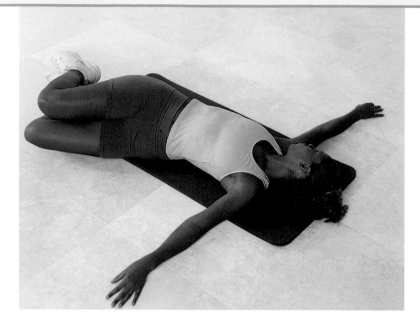

LAT STRETCH

To stretch the latissimus dorsi (the large back muscle), keep your hips down and walk your hands to one side and then the other. Make sure your head stays between your elbows.

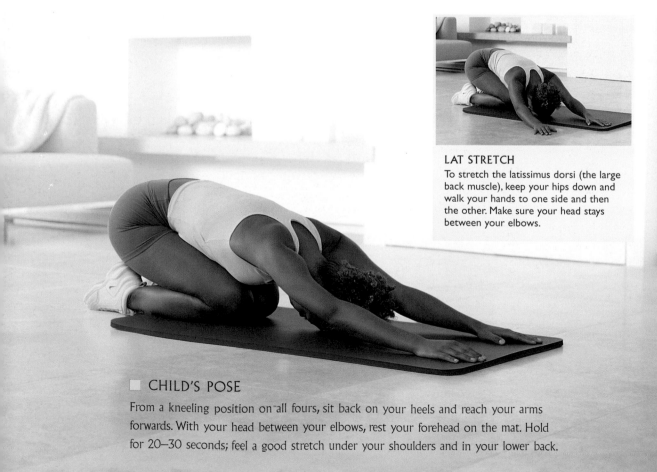

☐ CHILD'S POSE

From a kneeling position on all fours, sit back on your heels and reach your arms forwards. With your head between your elbows, rest your forehead on the mat. Hold for 20–30 seconds; feel a good stretch under your shoulders and in your lower back.

■ CAT STRETCH

Kneel on all fours, with your hands under your shoulders, fingers pointing straight ahead, and your knees under your hips. Round your back towards the ceiling, letting your head drop forwards. Reverse the position by bringing your head up and arching your lower back so that your spine curves the opposite way. If you have a touchy lower back, just bring the spine into neutral flat back position without arching it. Repeat 3 times each way.

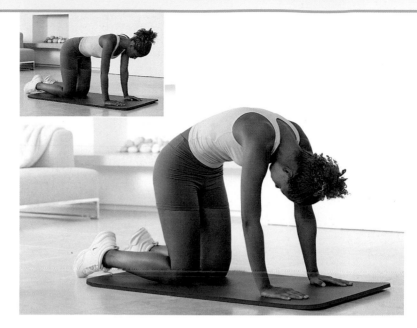

■ DOWNWARD FACING DOG

From the kneeling position, tuck your toes under and straighten your legs. Extend your arms fully and slowly reach up and back with your hips as you roll through your feet, pressing your heels towards the mat. Keep lengthening through the spine. Drop your head between your elbows. Feel the stretch in your spine, shoulders, hamstrings, and calf muscles. Hold the stretch for 20–30 seconds.

BENT KNEES
If your hamstrings are tight, keep your knees bent. Do not force your heels to touch the mat.

keep shoulders down

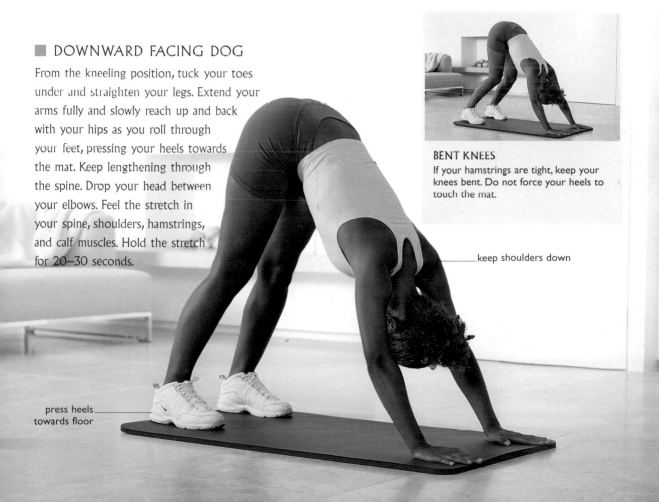

press heels
towards floor

THE MAJOR MUSCLE GROUPS

This programme covers all the major muscle groups and gives you a well-rounded, full-body workout. Performing one set of 12–15 reps of each exercise should take you about 30 minutes, once you learn the exercises. The less you rest between exercises, the more intense the workout.

Start with standing exercises for the lower body

Pause to stretch

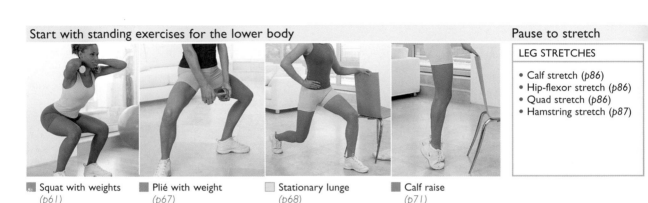

LEG STRETCHES
• Calf stretch (*p86*)
• Hip-flexor stretch (*p86*)
• Quad stretch (*p86*)
• Hamstring stretch (*p87*)

■ Squat with weights
(*p61*)

■ Plié with weight
(*p67*)

☐ Stationary lunge
(*p68*)

■ Calf raise
(*p71*)

Continue with floor work for the upper body

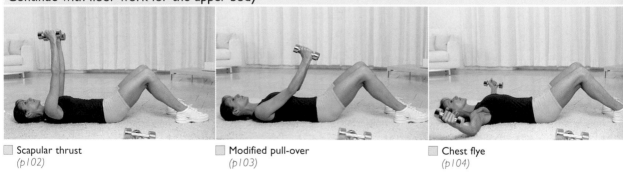

☐ Scapular thrust
(*p102*)

☐ Modified pull-over
(*p103*)

☐ Chest flye
(*p104*)

Finish with a series of core-body exercises

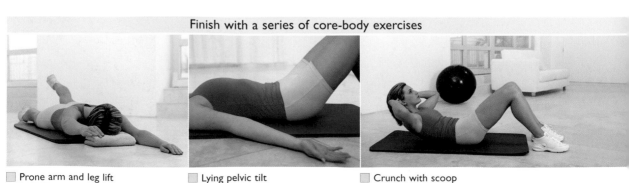

☐ Prone arm and leg lift
(*p136*)

☐ Lying pelvic tilt
(*p50*)

☐ Crunch with scoop
(*p129*)

TRAINING GUIDELINES

- Remember to warm up (pp32–37) before you start exercising and to stretch out after working the muscles.
- Use proper body alignment and good form.
- Start gently and avoid pain.
- Gradually increase the intensity.

- Always rest one day in between working the same muscle groups.
- The colour code indicates the level of skill required to perform the exercise:

  ☐ Beginner   ■ Intermediate   ■ Advanced

Move to standing exercises for the upper body

Go to the floor

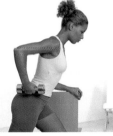

☐ One-arm row
(p94)

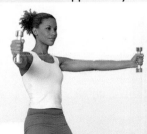

☐ Standing front raise
(p110)

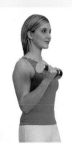

☐ Alternating biceps curl
(p116)

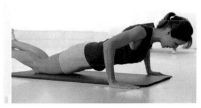

■ Half press-up
(p44)

Turn over for back work

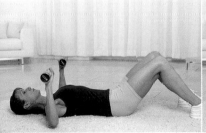

☐ Chest press
(p105)

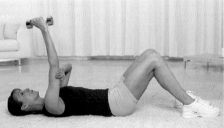

☐ Lying triceps extension
(p105)

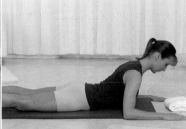

☐ Prone back extension
(p48)

Don't forget to cool down

COOLING DOWN STRETCHES

- Full-body stretch (p146)
- The bridge (p146)
- Low-back stretch (p147)
- Spinal twists (p148)
- Cat stretch (p149)
- Downward facing dog (p149)

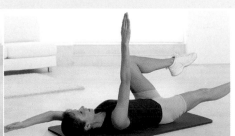

☐ Side crunch
(p130)

■ Dead bug
(p134)

IMPROVING POSTURE

Many people are concerned about their posture, particularly if they have a tendency to hunch forward. This programme strengthens the muscles of the midback to lift the chest, the glutes to support the back, and the core muscles to maintain an upright position. To balance your workout, I have added the Wall Press-Up to target the chest and shoulder.

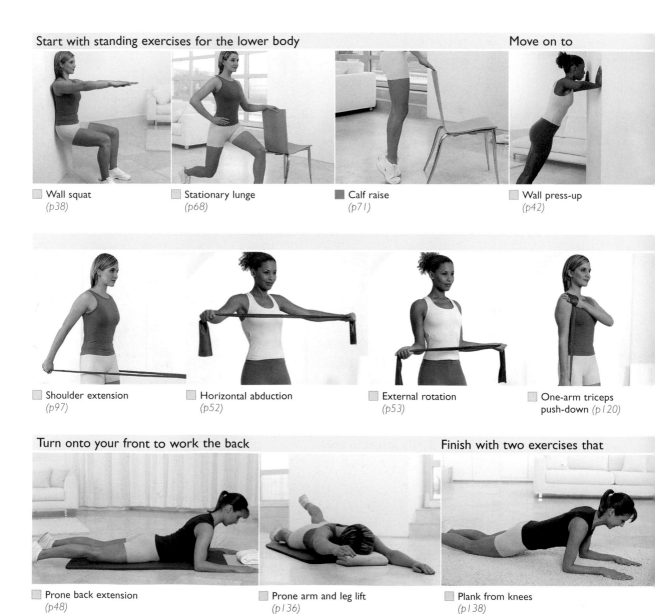

Start with standing exercises for the lower body   Move on to

☐ Wall squat
(p38)

☐ Stationary lunge
(p68)

☐ Calf raise
(p71)

☐ Wall press-up
(p42)

☐ Shoulder extension
(p97)

☐ Horizontal abduction
(p52)

☐ External rotation
(p53)

☐ One-arm triceps
push-down (p120)

Turn onto your front to work the back   Finish with two exercises that

☐ Prone back extension
(p48)

☐ Prone arm and leg lift
(p136)

☐ Plank from knees
(p138)

TRAINING GUIDELINES

- Remember to warm up (*pp32–37*) before you start exercising and to stretch out after working the muscles.
- Use proper body alignment and good form.
- Start gently and avoid pain.
- Gradually increase the intensity.

- Always rest one day in between working the same muscle groups.
- The colour code indicates the level of skill required to perform the exercise:

☐ Beginner ◼ Intermediate

standing exercises for the upper body

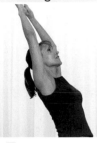 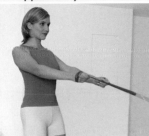 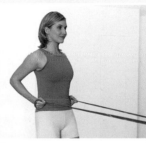 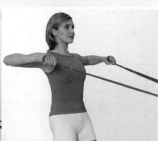

◼ Sun salutation (*p47*) ☐ Scapular retraction (*p96*) ☐ Lat row (*p96*) ☐ Upper-back row (*p97*)

Go to the floor to work the lower body, then move on to the core-body work exercises

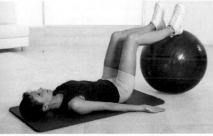 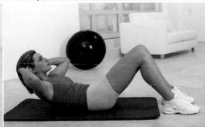 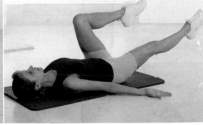

☐ Raised glute squeeze (*p76*) ☐ Crunch with scoop (*p129*) ◼ Alternating kicks (*p133*)

work your core stability

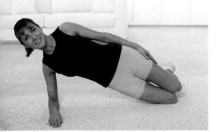

☐ Side plank from knees (*p140*)

Don't forget to cool down

COOLING DOWN STRETCHES

- Child's pose (*p148*)
- Lat stretch (*p148*)
- Cat stretch (*p149*)
- Downward facing dog (*p149*)
- Chest stretch (*p54*)
- Upper-back stretch (*p54*)
- Lat stretch (*p55*)

- Torso stretch (*p55*)
- Posterior-deltoid stretch (*p123*)
- Anterior-deltoid stretch (*p123*)
- Triceps stretch (*p123*)

BALANCE AND COORDINATION

When you are ready for more advanced work, these exercises will really challenge your strength, balance, and coordination in a new way. Before you begin these exercises, you should have strong core muscles and good control of handling your own body weight. Being able to do this programme is a real accomplishment.

Start with standing exercises for the lower body   Move on to the upper body

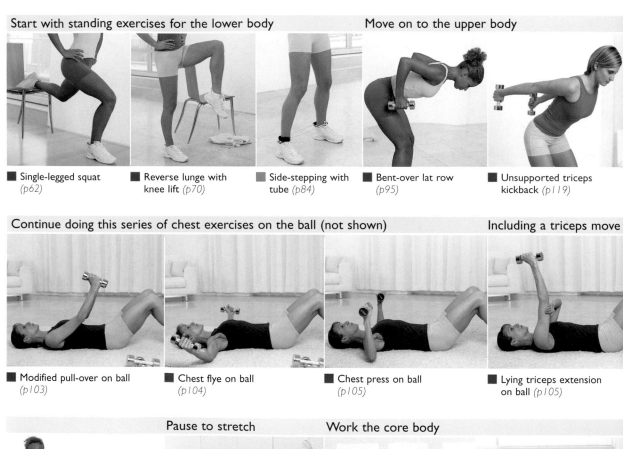

■ Single-legged squat *(p62)*

■ Reverse lunge with knee lift *(p70)*

■ Side-stepping with tube *(p84)*

■ Bent-over lat row *(p95)*

■ Unsupported triceps kickback *(p119)*

Continue doing this series of chest exercises on the ball (not shown)   Including a triceps move

■ Modified pull-over on ball *(p103)*

■ Chest flye on ball *(p104)*

■ Chest press on ball *(p105)*

■ Lying triceps extension on ball *(p105)*

Pause to stretch   Work the core body

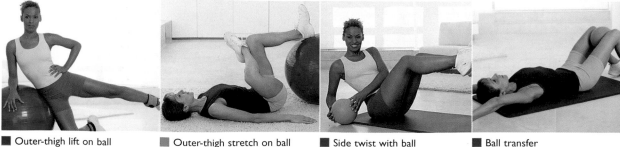

■ Outer-thigh lift on ball *(p81)*

■ Outer-thigh stretch on ball *(p89)*

■ Side twist with ball *(p131)*

■ Ball transfer *(p135)*

TRAINING GUIDELINES

- Remember to warm up (*pp32–37*) before you start exercising and to stretch out after working the muscles.
- Use proper body alignment and good form.
- Start gently and avoid pain.
- Gradually increase the intensity.

- Always rest one day in between working the same muscle groups.
- The colour code indicates the level of skill required to perform the exercise:

  ☐ Intermediate   ■ Advanced

Work on the ball for the back, then the chest and the arms

Lie on the ball for chest work

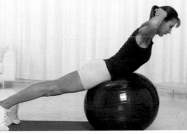

■ Back extension on ball (*p49*)

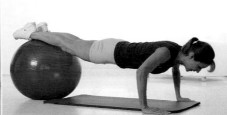

■ Full press-up on ball (*p15*)

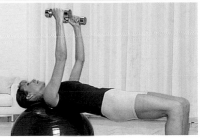

■ Scapular thrust on ball (*p102*)

Go to the floor for lower-body work

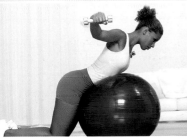

■ "Ys" and "Ts" on ball (*p115*)

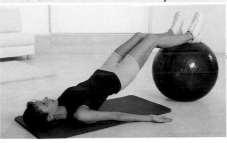

■ Ball bridge (*p77*)

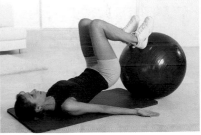

■ Leg curl on ball (*p77*)

Kneel to work the back

Don't forget to cool down

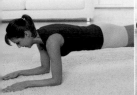

■ Full plank (*p139*)

■ Side plank from feet (*p141*)

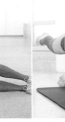

■ Kneeling arm and leg lift (*p136*)

STRETCHES

- Child's pose (*p148*)
- Lat stretch (*p148*)
- Cat stretch (*p149*)
- Downward facing dog (*p149*)
- Stretch on ball (*p87*)
- Sun salutation (*p47*)
- Triceps stretch (*p123*)

TARGETING THE TROUBLE SPOTS

This programme emphasizes all the well-known trouble spots: buttocks, thighs, waist, belly, and upper arms. It is a great workout to do if you are approaching the summer vacation and want to look good in swimwear, shorts, or skimpy tops. Give yourself at least a month of doing the exercises three times a week and you should see results.

Start with standing exercises for the lower body · Move on to

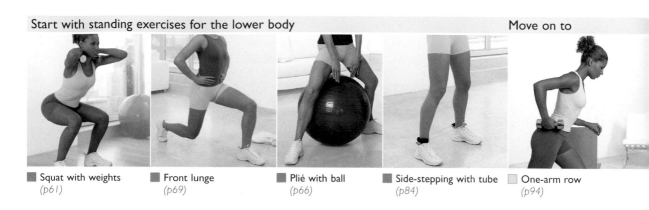

- ◼ Squat with weights (p61)
- ◼ Front lunge (p69)
- ◼ Plié with ball (p66)
- ◼ Side-stepping with tube (p84)
- ◻ One-arm row (p94)

Pause to stretch

UPPER BODY STRETCHES

- Triceps stretch (p123)
- Biceps and forearm stretch (p123)

Go to the floor to work your lower body

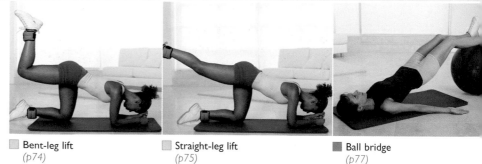

- ◻ Bent-leg lift (p74)
- ◻ Straight-leg lift (p75)
- ◼ Ball bridge (p77)

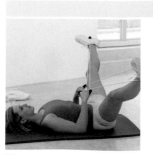

- ◼ Scissors with tubes (p85)

Pause to stretch

LOWER BODY STRETCHES

- Hamstring stretch (p147)
- Inner-thigh stretch (p88)
- Outer-thigh stretch (p89)
- Glute stretch (p89)

Work the core body

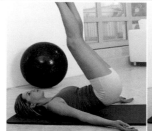
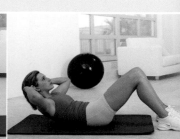

- ◼ Reverse crunch (p128)
- ◻ Crunch with scoop (p129)

TRAINING GUIDELINES

- Remember to warm up (pp32–37) before you start exercising and to stretch out after working the muscles.
- Use proper body alignment and good form.
- Start gently and avoid pain.
- Gradually increase the intensity.

- Always rest one day in between working the same muscle groups.
- The colour code indicates the level of skill required to perform the exercise:
  ☐ Beginner   ◪ Intermediate   ■ Advanced

standing work for the upper body

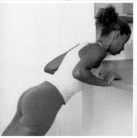 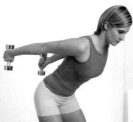 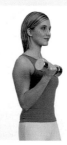 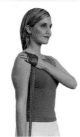 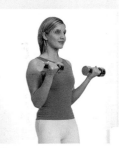

■ Diagonal press-up (p43)

■ Unsupported triceps kickback (p119)

☐ One-arm triceps push-down (p120)

☐ Alternating biceps curl (p116)

■ Biceps "21s" (p117)

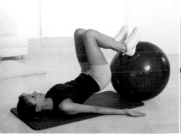 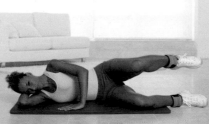 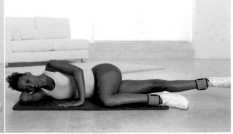

■ Leg curl on ball (p77)

☐ Outer-thigh lift (p80)

☐ Inner-thigh lift (p81)

After Dead Bug, stretch out your body

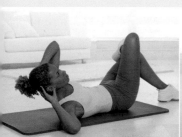 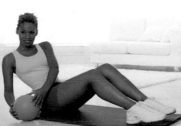 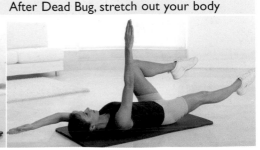

☐ Side crunch (p130)

■ Side twist with ball (p131)

■ Dead bug (p134); finish with Full-body stretch (p146)

INDEX

RESOURCES

Joan Pagano Fitness Group
401 East 89th Street (no. 2M)
New York, NY 10128, USA
Email: info@joanpaganofitness.com
www.joanpaganofitness.com

EQUIPMENT
I recommend that you order your equipment from a mailorder company. In the US, I use:
Fitness Wholesale®
Tel: 001–330–929–7227
email: fw@fwonline.com
www.fitnesswholesale.com
For free weights; ankle weights; a range of fitness balls, including stability balls; a stability-ball pump; tubes; mats; and stretch bands. They supply worldwide.

Best Priced Products, Inc.
Tel: 001–914–345–3800
email: FrontDesk@Bpp2.com
www.Bpp2.com
For wrist and ankle weights with a long touch-fastener tail.

Topaz Medical, Ltd.
email: info@topazusa.com
www.topazusa.com.
For MediBalls (gel-filled medicine balls).

For the UK
Totally Fitness
Tel: 020–7467–5925
email: sales@totallyfitness.com
www.r2b.com
For free weights, stability balls, stretch bands, resistance tubes.

Newitt & Co Ltd
Tel: 01904–468551
email: sales@newitts.com
www.newitts.com
For medicine balls, free weights, ankle weights, and stretch bands.

Sissel UK Limited
Tel: 01422–885433
email: info@sisseluk.com
www.sisseluk.com
For thick gym mat, stability balls (the Sissel Fitbox), and stretch bands.

National Osteoporosis Society (NOS)
Camerton, Bath BA2 0PJ
Tel: 01761–471771 (general enquiries)
Helpline (medical): 0845–4500230
email: info@nos.org.uk
www.nos.org.uk

For Australia
Elite Fitness Equipment
Tel: (In Australia only) 1800–622–644
email: info@elitefitness.com.au
www.elitefitness.com.au

Fernwood Women's Health Club
National office
Tel: (03) 5443–4555
Phone a club: 13–33–76
www.fernwoodfitness.com.au

Osteoporosis Australia
Level 1, 52 Parramatta Road Forest Lodge, NSW 2037
Tel: (02) 9518–8140
www.osteoporosis.org.au

ACKNOWLEDGMENTS

AUTHOR'S ACKNOWLEDGMENTS

Grateful acknowledgments to all who helped shape this book: Jenny Jones, my brilliant editor, creative muse, and eternally patient advisor; and the rest of the DK team: Mary-Clare Jerram, Sara Robin, and Gillian Roberts for their warmth, kindness, and professional expertise. My clients for their loyalty over the years and for their generosity of spirit. My personal support team: James, for his unconditional love, and for always being there with an open mind; Lucy, my sister, my coach, for her inspired teaching; Susan, for her big heart and expert knowledge of anatomy; CJ, for her courage to explore new frontiers and share the path; Haila, mentor and agent of change, for being a guiding force in my career. My colleagues at Marymount Manhattan College, for all they have taught me.

PUBLISHER'S ACKNOWLEDGMENTS

Dorling Kindersley would like to thank photographer Graham Atkins-Hughes (studio) and his assistant, Raul Fernandez; and Russell Sadur (gym) and his assistant, Emil Stevenson; models Yasmin Phillips, Kirsty Spence, and Sally Way; Victoria Barnes, for models' hair and makeup; stylist Liz Hippisley; Philip Wilson for the illustrations; Margaret Parrish for editorial assistance; Lynn Bresler for the index; and Sonia Charbonnier for all her DTP support. Special thanks to Barclay Harvey, Karen Edmunds, and Michael Arnold at Reebok Sports Club, Canary Wharf, London; The White Company for throws, towels, and cushions (www.thewhiteco.com or tel: 0870 900 9555), and The Chair Company for chairs (www.thechair.co.uk or tel. 020 7091 1155). All images © DK Images. For more information see www.dkimages.com

ABOUT THE AUTHOR

JOAN PAGANO is certified by the American College of Sports Medicine (ACSM) in health/fitness instruction. ACSM credentials provide the very best measure of competence as a professional. Since 1988, she has worked as a personal fitness trainer on Manhattan's Upper East Side, New York, providing professional guidance and support to people at all levels of fitness. Through her work she has created hundreds of training programmes for individuals, groups, fitness facilities, schools, hospitals, and corporations.

Today, Joan manages her own staff of fitness specialists, who work together as Joan Pagano Fitness Group. She is also Director of the Marymount Manhattan College Personal Fitness Trainer Certification Programme, and a member of the IDEA Personal Trainer Committee, an organization that supports health and fitness professionals worldwide with education, career development, and leadership. She is also a nationally recognized provider of continuing education courses for fitness trainers.

Joan's knowledge of women's health issues evolved naturally from her work. Women trust Joan to guide them through periods of physical transition, such as pregnancy and childbirth, recovery from surgery, or when fighting disease. As fitness consultant to SHARE (a breast cancer support group), she has worked with breast cancer survivors since 1992. Their concerns about menopause prompted Joan to study how exercise could help manage the side effects of this stage in life, and, in particular, how exercise could help fight osteoporosis. Now Joan is recognized by the industry as a leading authority on exercise programme design strategies for osteoporosis.